Copyright© 2019
Published by: Zeno & Zeno Publishing, LLC 445 N. Main St., #1702 Suffolk, Virginia 23434, www.ZandZPublishing.com
Edited by Simon Timm
Cover & Interior Illustration: Claudia Rose, Ph.D.
Photographer: Eric Clark
Interior Design: Andrea Huff
LCCN: 2019908549

All rights reserved. No part of this book may be reproduced in whole or in part or transmitted by any means electronic, mechanical, photocopy, recording; nor may it be stored in a retrieval system, transmitted, or otherwise copied for public or private use, other than "fair use," as in brief quotations in articles and reviews, without prior written permission.

The author does not dispense medical advice nor encourage the use of any technique as a form of medical treatment without the advice of a physician. Information of a general nature is offered to assist the reader in their quest of emotional and spiritual well-being. Results are the sole responsibility of the reader, not the author and/or publisher. The names and identifying characteristics of certain individuals referenced in this publication have been changed. This publication is sold with the understanding that neither the author or publisher are qualified mental health professionals (QMHP). If the reader requires such advice or services a competent physician or licensed qualified mental health profession should be consulted.

No warranty is made with respect to the accuracy or completeness of the information contained herein, and both the author and publisher specifically disclaim any responsibility for any liability, loss, or risk, personal or otherwise, which is incurred as a consequence, directly or indirectly, of the use and application of any of the contents of this book.

This book deals with sensitive subjects and may evoke strong emotion for some readers.

Other books by PerCilla Zeno

Visit:

www.ZandZpublishing.com

Percilla Zeno

I AM *Healing*

7 Secrets to Wellness and Self-Care

"Dear Self,
There's a garden of love within us.
It's the place where you and I meet and understand each other more,
spend time with each other more, love and forgive each other more.
So, take off your KOOL and stay in tune for a while or forever.
Either way, I promise to heal you."
Love Always,
Your Higher Self
- PerCilla
#QuotePerCillaZ

Dedication

This book is dedicated to my Higher Power, Ancestors and spiritual guides, who continuously look after me, are connected to me, speak to me, and lead me directly to my highest and best. I'm excited to see whom these gifts will touch and where these gifts will take me. I am so grateful.

To my loving husband, Luis—for being my soul mate and best friend, for believing in me, giving me what I've needed and how I needed it, even when you didn't understand it; for offering a space in time where I could share my greatest hopes, dreams, and illusions (fears). Thank you for the love you continue to give me and the brilliant thoughts you share that make me fall in love with you all over again each day.

How much do I love thee?
Deeper than the deepest ocean
and farther than the eye can see…

To my mother Jacquie—for your gentle nudges during the noise, teaching me to finish what I start and to never give up; showing me when to be quiet and when to fight like hell. A part of you had to die so that we, your children, could live. I understand it was a choice. Thank you for choosing us. I am so proud to call you my mother.

To Dej, Bear, DLo, Vanni—*my children*—for the beauty in each one of you and for being four of my reasons to be better and to evolve daily. There is no such thing as a perfect person, but there is a true perfection in love and healing. I couldn't have made it this far without each of you. Love, Ma

To David Rudolph, Sr.—you are and will always be an *amazing* father. I will forever be grateful for the children we share. Your name will never be erased from our hearts.

To my grandmothers Mittie C. Riley-Williams and Elizabeth Redfearn-Reid, both of whose comforting presences are forever with me.

Mr. & Mrs. Stephen Temko – for being the attorney and wife that was selfless, courageous and just all-around descent human beings on this planet. I will never forget the love and kindness you've shown us.

Last but not least, to my son, 'Lil Dave—like your birth, your transcendence from this earthly realm to the next continues to be an internal and eternal gift. At birth, you gave me the gift of knowing motherhood, love, compassion, strength and understanding. Your exit brought the gift and true meaning of motherhood, love, compassion, strength, and understanding, as well as forgiveness. You were needed here, and now you're needed there to do bigger and better things on a higher plane. My harmony and inner peace are living proof that you had to be a part of something larger than ourselves. Your parting was never a loss; on the contrary, my willingness to let go of the sorrow has allowed me to gain more light, more oneness, and more wisdom than I could ever have imagined.

For this, I am so grateful to Spirit. For this, I am so grateful for you. Thank you, my precious son.

Table of Contents

Preface: 1
  Where Did My Flow Go? Restoring Your Energy Stream
Chapter 1 13
  Secret #1: Superheroes Don't Need Self-Care, But You Do!
Chapter 2 27
  Secret #2: From the Cover Up to the Cure
Chapter 3 37
  Secret #3: Fear the Cycle
Chapter 4 49
  Secret #4: When You Forgive, You Live!
Chapter 5 61
  Secret #5: The Process of Sifting
Chapter 6 73
  Secret #6: Forward…Growing…Evolving!
Chapter 7 85
  Secret #7: Making the Most of Missteps & Mistakes
Bonus 97
  The Energy that Flows from Within – *Chakra Doors*
Final Thoughts .... Pg 115
Resources .... Pg 133

Where Did My Flow Go? Restoring Your Energy Stream

"Being mindful of your needs means loving yourself enough to effect a positive change."
– PerCilla Zeno, The Healing Partner

IMAGINE if you will that you are floating down a crystal-clear river of healing. Its tranquil, sparkling current is relaxing and soothing… bringing a sense of calm to every part of you. Nevertheless, negative feelings still creep in, and all of the negative feelings you are experiencing on a minute-to-minute basis drop into the river, instantly depositing bits of pollution and trash.

At every moment you feel stressed, or anxious, or down… every time you endure an ounce of pain, another bit of pollution slips into the stream. The pollution not only dirties and clogs up the watercourse but grows thick enough to slow your progress, making your passage more and more difficult.

Meanwhile, everyone expects you to go on about your life and keep moving forward. So, you go to work. You care for your family.

You contribute to your neighborhood, religious community, and friendships. You participate in life, doing your very best not to let on that you feel increasingly clogged, stuck, overwhelmed, and completely trapped—and you cannot see or feel your way out.

Now, let me ask you a question: while you are taking care of everyone else, who the hell is taking care of you? When *no one* is taking care of you (not even *you*), then the flow of your life starts to clog up. Your stress, worry, and pain build up more and more…every moment of every day. These feelings add thick layers of fear and doubt that further pollute the river of your life and your ability to make progress and move forward to your own hopes and dreams in the physical, mental, emotional, and spiritual realms of your journey.

All of this toxicity makes aligning to your deepest self, your *I AM*, seem almost impossible. You might even wonder what forward movement would ultimately mean for you after a while. Well, the simple truth is that *you* are the forward movement! Your dreams, your personal, professional, and financial goals…your entire life! And your "*I AM*" waits for you to align the inner you with the outer you. When that alignment happens, you learn how to get through life and clear the blockages of emotional, physical, and mental ailments. You learn to let go of the resistance and accept the forward flow, despite all obstacles. You learn how to take care of you.

Forward movement is the freedom to "be well" in every area. Being well takes the shape of being self-loving, being present and progressive, being healed and healing, being connected to your Higher Source, and/or being free to just *be*—and it's possible to begin the process right now, wherever you are in life. When you have aligned your energy properly, you will find that moving forward into the flow of life will move you towards the highest and best expression of who you truly are. That is your *I AM*. It's that part of you that gives hope during the most difficult thoughts and challenges. What do you face day-to-day? Are you feeling the flow, or are you stuck?

Listen to me carefully: There is hope! No matter what your current day-to-day contains, there is more to life than merely overcoming hurdles. There is more to life than just gritting your teeth and bearing through the freaking unbearable. There is an internal and eternal beauty of harmony and love…peace, balance, and yes, bliss, that comes from being properly aligned within the mind, body, and spirit—and flowing forward on the journey to your highest and best self.

How do I know this is possible? Because I've experienced what it feels like to be in the place of depletion of mind, body, and spirit. I've been sad, hurt, and full of pain, fearful, doubting, and anxious. I've been depressed, full of sickness and dis-ease. I've thought the darkest thoughts while wrapped up in chains of my own guilt, fear, anger and vengeance. All the while, I had the audacity to pretend I was living my best life.

In those days I'd felt stuck in my life for so long that I almost forgot I was flowing anywhere. Furthermore, when I was living my unhealthy, disconnected life, I endured the worst possible thing that could happen to anyone: my son died. Dropping me into the place of surreal despair, this traumatic loss threw me off balance even more. I was completely and utterly fearful about life moving forward and at a loss for the answers that I needed.

While working through the dark days that followed the death of my son, I at long last experienced a sudden epiphany. In a moment's flash I was instantly able to grasp the reality that my life's priority and responsibility should, first and foremost, be me. As I took ownership of this fact, I began to understand that if I didn't move on this new understanding *now* I would miss opportunity after opportunity that lay ahead on the journey to create the life I'd always wanted.

Honestly, I wasn't even aware of *what* all I wanted at the time, but I knew I wanted a change. Cast into the reality that no tomorrow is promised to us, and that I was letting life happen *to me*, I welcomed the new understanding that life happens to *be me*.

Now I began mentally telling myself a more empowering story from a truer belief system: I AM *clarity.* I AM *peace.* I AM *from a limitless Source of energy that has no area of lack in all areas of life, and* I AM *so much more....*

Nonetheless, how was I going to get free physically from where I was and move into a healthy state of being well, doing well, and authentically radiating those higher (vibrational) thoughts so that I could attract the same type of experiences back into my life? How would I arrive at a place where I could be still and listen to the songs of my life challenges—without killing the best part of my urge to dance over any small triumphs?

It was clear at that point that tapping into my usual sources of motivation and inspiration wasn't going to be enough. I was too profoundly restricted by the pollution and bits of trash that were clogging my watercourse. I had to move, or succumb to my *stuckness* in grief, anger, fear, hiding, and heaviness, which were rapidly creeping in and halting my progress.

Something had to give. Slowly moving forward from my life trials and now devastating loss, I began to accept that life isn't just about surviving loss and pain. Life is worth investing in on a much deeper, more committed and intentional level, using our mindful ability to transcend pain and be present in life.

Mindfully, I had to take the steps to embrace a new way of thinking. Simply put, it was this: *I am no good to anyone if I am not lovingly good to me. So, to hell with anything that stands between me and that rich, full, healthy, loving life I was born to live, especially before giving it—and all of myself—away to others.* Sounds *self-ish* right? Read on.

Decide to Move Forward, and then Do It!

As I said, the rise from the depths of grieving my loss was still a continuing process, but after my epiphany it didn't take me a long time to act on my new and higher plane of mindfulness. I was now fully open and willing to move—and be moved— even a small distance farther. My dreams were now pulling me up and beckoning me forward.

So, one of the first active decisions that I made in the process of my own healing and building the life I wanted was to pursue weight-loss surgery. I had thought about it for a few years. It was not a quick or easy decision, especially considering the physical and financial demands the choice would place on me.

Nevertheless, the surgery gave me the jump-start I needed to dive into the work of healing and flourishing, in a way I knew I was capable of healing and flourishing.

What holds us back from acting on our inner knowledge that more is possible in our lives? I think that when we forget to make ourselves a priority and overlook aligning the *I AM* within us, we get caught up in routines.

Living becomes a cycle where there just isn't time to do those things that move us toward our dreams and into who we truly are. We feel like we're stuck, holding our breath until we can get a free moment to imagine what our life could be. And before you know it, we have lost sight of our dreams—and ourselves.

Meanwhile, a special warm and fuzzy place is made for others to breathe easy. The question is: How could *you* breathe easy, and flow forward into your highest and best life, while not disregarding the needs of those around you? This is not selfishness, but *selfhood*.

First of all, exhale. Don't give up before you start. The time is now. If you've picked up this book, you know in your soul that your free moment is this one, right here, right now. Time is not going to get any *free-er* in the future, and your *I AM* is ready and willing to lend you the strength you already possess to clear out all the litter and to wrap yourself up in the flow of self-healing and self-care *today*.

In these pages you will hear me reference your *I AM*. Though you may find the term odd or unfamiliar, try to picture the uppermost loving peak of expression within that desires to befriend and care for you. What is the *I AM* within us?

The *I AM* is the highest and best part of you, the part that wants the highest and best for you.

The *I AM* within you is that which awaits the willingness to freely remove the congested, blocked energy and tension that binds you.

Again, the *I AM* is the inner you, the non-physical you…that innocent, loving, courageous, exposed, tranquil, forgiving, true, honest, and most beautiful you. This is who you were before you were birthed. Anything else is an illusion.

The *I AM* knows how to process your stillness.

The *I AM* knows how to bring you inner peace, love, and harmony.

Your will to align the energy from the *I AM* to the physical is what brings you to wellness.

"The Healing Partner" Work

Sometimes your mind is so congested with the smog of racing thoughts and consuming fear that your *I AM* is silenced. The more the mental congestion, the heavier you become. But your *I AM* never leaves you. Instead, it waits for you to align the inner you with the physical you. It waits for the energy and strength that is free-flowing, unhindered, and unobstructed to move you to action.

In this book I'll share with you my stories of self-healing. I'll provide thoughts on how you can become more mindful of your self-healing and self-care needs, along with assessments to help you get there. At the end of each chapter, you will find "The Healing Partner" personal work section. In it, I will offer a number of things you can implement in your life today to improve your own ability to heal. This section will also educate you, at a beginner's level, on the different energy areas within your body that are in need of healing. Each "Healing Partner" section will include the following:

◊ An Affirmation – Reaffirming what you already know and who you truly are.

◊ An Acknowledgement – For acknowledging the stress you carry and what it may be connected to internally.

◊ "The Healing Partner" Thoughts – Tools, exercises, and actions you can put in place now to jump-start your self-healing and self-care process.

◊ An Attunement – To help you become more aware

and bring into harmony the parts of the Human Energy Field (HEF) affected during distressing life experiences or in life recovery.

There are seven chakras, also known as "wheels of energy," within us, through which the energy flows. When blockages occur or energy is compromised, it's important to know where they are. Energy blockages affect our mental, physical, emotional, and spiritual planes. Energy imbalances keep us stuck and carry pain, *dis-ease*, jealousy, discomfort, and a host of other unwanted sufferings. But you *can* work with them and gain freedom.

Energy Healing: What It is, and Isn't

Now, if you're thinking that the human energy field (HEF) is as about as real as global warming and that *both* are complete hogwash, rubbish, or just utter *bullsh*t*—I'm sorry to tell you, but it is a scientific fact that global warming is very real. And the human energy field is no different. It's a measurable scientific reality.

Energy Healing (an alternative medicine) is increasingly being used in hospitals in America today (see references) as a complementary therapy to traditional medicine. Be it oncology patient support, pre-operative and post-operative recovery, and/or with an extended variety of patients, energy healing has been shown to be of benefit, helping the body to release stress and recuperate more quickly. It can also be useful for reducing stress levels in clients in recovery from eating disorders, agoraphobia, substance abuse, and other life issues of "stuckness."

Doctors and nurses also participate in energy healing in order to decrease their stress levels. I *know*, because the certifications I hold allow me to work with these very people—doctors, nurses, and regular clients, inside and outside of the hospital. If you are open to this new field of knowledge in human functioning, it holds the possibility of opening so many doors for you and may take you down many new pathways toward optimal health.

Being mindful of your needs means loving yourself enough to effect a positive change. It means you believe you deserve to heal and clear the energy pathways within yourself in order to embrace a better, healthier, more balanced, and more peaceful life. Even if you don't know how to achieve those things right now, that's OK! We all start somewhere, and we are each a work in progress.

Remember, you are not alone. You never *were* alone; you just didn't know it! You may feel like you're walking this road in solitude; like nobody understands your struggles and difficulties, or that nobody cares. Well, *I do,* and in this book I hope you will find the truth: that there are other caring souls. We are all connected, even if our stories aren't the same.

The first step on the path toward aligning your *I AM* with the light of love and peace is to pursue self-healing. For those of you who may think that because of what you've done, or what was *done to you,* you don't deserve respect or harmony or wholeness, this just isn't true. For those who may think everyone deserves harmony, love, balance, and peace, but feel you are just semi-connected to that truth, that's OK, too. Keep moving!

Your Healing Partner Is Here

I wrote this book to show people like you—*people like me*—that there is hope and that we each hold within ourselves the power to change. I want to convince you of that. The journey and personal confessions I share will, I hope, be the catalyst needed to spark an epiphany in you, too—and allow you to see new possibilities for your life.

Often what we really need is a friend on our journey, a *healing partner* in our lifeboat. A little guidance never hurt anybody—especially when it's helping us transcend painful stuckness in areas that we usually struggle with in silence. That's what I'm offering to you: the opportunity to see the *victor* in your silent struggle and to open your heart to receive the courage to allow the healing pathway that lies before you to draw you forward. And I would be honored to be your Healing Partner.

Now, *exhale!* It's time to awaken your *I AM,* to greet and reacquaint yourself with the real you—the *victorious* you within!

—PerCilla Zeno

I Am...

Secret #1
Superheroes Don't Need Self-Care, but you do!

"Warning: Your pride will always try to stop you from asking for help! See that as a yellow sign, and not a red one."
— PerCilla, "The Healing Partner"

I used to think I was Superwoman, so much so that I even bragged about it! If there was a crisis, I'd take control of everything and everyone involved in it. I'd take on whatever problems my family, my friends, my business, my clients had—making sure to find a solution or fix what I felt needed fixing. Yet while I was making sure everybody else was good, I wasn't taking care of me, at all, or seeing my delusion of having everything under control.

I was what you might call a "presser." I'd do what needed to be done and press on or press it down deep within (no matter my need or pain). It took a while before the result of that faulty thinking and daily practice reared its pretty little head. And when it did, I quickly understood that I most certainly was not Superwoman. What it took for me to understand this, to be completely honest with you, was a genuine nervous breakdown.

Overwhelmed by my inability to be perfect and strong at all times, I became very fearful, trusting no one outside of those I already knew. It got to the point where I didn't want to leave my room because I was afraid someone would hurt me. Make no mistake about it, the pressed-down emotions I had been harboring since I was a wee little thing were now bubbling over. I stayed in my bedroom all day long. And if I left at all, I would not go anywhere without my dogs.

What was happening in this emotional meltdown was that the hard things I'd endured as a child had begun to surface uncontrollably. One by one, they crept up like thieves in the night, and then strangled me. Intense pain in my upper back, and also panic attacks, began to grip me—and were especially likely to happen in small, tight spaces.

The event that triggered this initially was my reading the transcript from my father's court trial in January of 1991, in which he was sentenced to "life, plus twenty years." I honestly thought I was over the triggers from anything that had to do with my father. So much so that I allowed him to send his transcript to me to transfer to his lawyer.

I had no idea that my curiosity to know the details of what happened in his trial would result in my experiencing this overwhelming amount of fear. As I read through the account of charges against my father, I was hurled into a pit of painful memories—and I didn't know how to deal with them. This also became overwhelming for my husband, because I'd question his whereabouts every time he'd get up to do something as simple as use the restroom.

After several weeks of living in a state of fear, I finally realized that I had to do something about my situation. My hesitation to share what

I Am Healing - Secret #1

was going on inside me came from my pride in my own self-sufficiency. I was mortified of what my family, friends, and those who looked up to me would think if they found out I was weak now, and what people would say about me visiting a psychotherapist. You see, I was supposed to be the smart, pretty, strong "businesswoman who had it all together." That was my illusion and my reality!

Nonetheless, I couldn't very well live life locked up inside the four walls of my bedroom. I mustered enough courage to call my mother and my friend, and they were able to get me to go to a counselor.

Change Requires Courage

During my first visit I ended up talking to a beautiful lady who made me feel incredibly comfortable and safe. We talked about many things and, eventually, her questions began to shift toward my past. I answered them reluctantly, and with quick, short answers. She could tell I was nervous and handed me a book entitled *The Courage to Heal Workbook* by Laura Davis.

In the back of the book there were multiple blank pages, providing a space where I, the trauma victim, could write out what had happened to me. While I flipped through the pages, my counselor encouraged me to write whatever I could remember from the abuse I had experienced. The book sat on my nightstand collecting dust for quite a while.

For obvious reasons, and some less obvious, I didn't want to write in it. For one, I knew it wasn't going to be a "sit out by the pool with some jazz music and a cocktail while you sprinkle some thoughts on a page"—type of experience. No, I knew this was going to be a much greater challenge.

Pulling this pain up and out of me would make me rethink all the *shoulda, coulda, woulda's* in my life, and it would require mentally reliving all of the hurtful, horrible experiences I had been through. For a long time I knew it needed to be done for me to get free of fear.

When the therapist would check in with me about it, I'd give some lame-ass excuse about why I hadn't written anything in the book. The truth, however (and I knew it), was that as long as I held on to the pain deep inside of me, my heaviness and fear would remain and the *true me* (the *I AM*) would never emerge.

I was off and on in therapy that year, since I had no real commitment to my own healing. Eventually, on one sunny afternoon, I decided to pick up the book and write it all out. I was overwhelmed and tired of pretending that everything was OK. I needed to pull back internally and mentally regroup. So, I picked up an ink pen and wrote everything out in detail, as much as I could honestly remember.

I wrote and wrote, until all the painful memories that had been hidden away in my heart for years now lay before me in clear black and white. The wounds they represented finally were exposed to the open light of day. With tears falling from my face onto the pages of the workbook, I acknowledged their reality and the trauma and pain I had experienced.

I wrote about my father and the sexual abuse I endured from him…about my first abusive encounter with him at five years old, when he called me from the second floor of our home to come upstairs, pulling me away from the rest of the family as they were having breakfast, just so that he could move his hand past my robe, and slip his fingers past my underwear as he whispered, "Keep quiet; I love you, and if you tell anyone, I'll kill you."

I Am Healing – Secret #1

I wrote about how my father would frequently turn my childhood disobedience into an opportunity to get me behind closed doors, beat me with a belt, and stick his fingers in me, so that my screams would confuse those who heard them. I wrote about the woman, a family friend, who would calculate my nap time so that she could lure me into the bedroom and make me lie on top of her as she'd gyrate her hips. I wrote about watching my father beat my mother horribly, to the point where she was close to death. I wrote about the plan to flee with my mother to the other side of the country to get away from my father.

I wrote about the trauma, the bulimia, and my own addiction to sex as a preteen and young adult—and anything and everything else that had affected me—so that I could shovel out the pain within me and bury it in the workbook. With each stroke of the pen I was gaining freedom, and was no longer the *graveyard for the hurt,* where I had entombed my feelings and myself for decades. When I was done writing my story, I closed the book, and never opened those pages again.

This exercise, and the therapy I underwent to process the trauma, helped me to understand why I had become a people pleaser and Superwoman. It helped me to understand why I became fearful when I lost my superpowers. It helped me to start to heal from all of this, and heal from the self-rejection and suffering I had put myself through, as well.

The healing had at last been kick-started, and for this I gave myself credit, despite the amount of time it took me to finally put my good intentions into action and get through the writing exercise. I wish

I could tell you that I stayed with my healing work back then but, unfortunately, I had still not grasped that well-being really is attained little by little, day by day. It may begin with a one-time catalyst, but we have to maintain it daily.

Superwoman Gets Grounded

Taking up my pen and writing out my truth helped me realize that I don't have to try and be a superhero. That was a cover-up for the toxic shame I was subjected to in my youth. No, I'm not Superwoman. I'm a *tenacious* woman. I'm a passionate woman. I'm a loving woman. I have Superwoman tendencies. And hell, I would even go as far as to say that, with the right wig I could pull off that Superwoman look! However, the fact is that I'm not her—and as soon as I dropped the illusion of being a superhero, I began to be more grounded and more able to stay in tune with reality. It was official: the heaviness I had carried for decades was no longer *as* heavy, because I had begun the work that Superwoman never had to do, the work of getting real and being healed.

You see, fictional superheroes never need a mental health day, a mani-pedi, or even a girls' or boys' night out! They don't need rest and recreation, or self-care. But human beings do! So, we must drop the illusion of flawlessness and of limitless strength in order to be *grounded* enough to know when it's time to halt and seek out rejuvenation (if we're going to continue to move forward).

I've learned that sometimes taking a break—pulling back from life and caring for *you* for awhile—is essential for self-healing and proper human self-care. If we do not, we may be in danger of a full *systems breakdown*. The story above is an example from my own life where I was forced to pull back from "super-selfing" in order to ground and stabilize myself in a more reality-based way.

Pulling back is something we need to practice on a day to day basis,

I Am Healing - Secret #1

as well. We have to learn how to slow down and mentally regroup when we're feeling overwhelmed—and this isn't the same as surrendering in defeat. Taking a break to regroup in stressful times is actually a form of *taking control* and preventing long-term burnout.

Pulling Back to Flow Forward

So, when you're in the habit of super-selfing, how do you know when it's time to pull back? The first way is to pay very close attention to your own inner voice when you start to feel overwhelmed—you know, the one telling you that something's off, or that you need to take care of yourself. If you've never even heard that voice, or you've never listened to and heeded it in your life, then you may need a *big break* in order to learn to tune in and examine what is going on under the surface of your busyness and activities.

Maybe you just need to pull back a little in order to avoid burnout, because you're used to working and ignoring your self-care needs instead of dealing with the things you struggle with in silence. Being overwhelmed can be a significant drain on your physical, spiritual, mental, and emotional energy. And in moments of exhaustion, when you're not thinking clearly, you may be tempted to do a host of things your body or mind doesn't really need, rather than to address your real, deeper need (which is much too scary to think about).

It's easy to ignore the fact that you're getting to the point of physical exhaustion when you're wrapped up in anything and everything else but yourself. I am grateful for my kids, my husband, my home, my client sessions, my retreats and workshops, and just for being able to wake up every morning. Though, with that said, I still must make some time in my schedule to give my neurons a break, or just to "check-in" with myself, if I'm going to keep my goals for all these things I love—and *myself*—flowing down the stream of life with a healthy perspective.

At check-in time you're telling your to-do list, your life situations, and your negative emotions to halt. You're telling everything to *wait* just a minute while you take a step back, lay down whatever needs to be laid down, and regroup. When you pull back and look at the situation from another angle, you're sending the message to others, and showing yourself, that *you* matter, too, just as they do.

The solution to not being overwhelmed isn't merely resting your body. *Mental* exhaustion is just as damaging as running your body to the brink of passing out! So, coming to a complete halt in your problem-solving mind may be just the thing that is needed to gather your thoughts, rest your body, and let your mind (in quietness) reveal what your next steps towards fulfilling your life goals or needs should be.

Remember that by pulling back you are not failing. You're just flowing in a different direction, one that will lead you back to the mainstream of things. As you regroup in your mind and body, keep your sense of purpose intact. A significant shift in perspectives is that, when you find yourself tired and worn out or overwhelmed, take the time to get what you need, knowing you're not giving up, you're just giving back—to yourself. You are Refueling. You are Grounding. You are balancing yourself in a healthy way.

Many stressful situations seem like they need to be taken care of immediately. Sometimes they can even seem terrifying at that moment. But trust me, if the toilet isn't overflowing, it sure as hell can wait! Most situations can be put on hold for at least a few minutes while you catch your breath, pull back, and check within for direction.

It's important to have some regular, habitual coping strategies in place and to make self-healing and self-care a part of your everyday practice. There will be times when you are exhausted, but you will be surprised by your ability to balance your energy in moments like this when you habitually care for yourself. There's no way to prevent life from throwing stress your way, but you *can* control how you treat yourself during stressful times. I'm not only living proof, but I'm one of the many who've learned a new and better, more authentic way to live. The concepts shared with you here are a handy guide for just that!

"The Healing Partner" Work

Affirmation

I am grounded, sustained, nourished and let go of the stress of feeling that my basic needs are not being met in every area of my life.

Acknowledgement

Acknowledge any stress and issues with feeling secure to manifest your basic self-needs and check-in with yourself when feeling overwhelmed by life.

Attune

Root Chakra: This energy is located at the base of the spine. Clearing a blockage in the root chakra will assist with areas of *survival* (will to live), trust, security, and other areas. Depending on your unique situation, there are healers, exercises, and meditations that can assist with this. Do your research and find what fits best for you.

"The Healing Partner" Thoughts

Below are a few *in-the-moment* things you can do to provide self-care in times of overwhelming stress. Some may sound similar, some new—and small adjustments for different situations or personality types are often all that's needed to make a solution work. Not every tip will work in every case, so use your best judgment. *What's best for you?*

1. Relaxation and restoration: Acquire some energy medicine from a healing touch practitioner or apprentice such as an HTP/HTP-A). Soak your body in a long, relaxing bath, or receive a massage. You can do one or all of these activities. They each put you in a different state of relaxation and restoration.

2. Take a trip: Whether it's on a plane, train, automobile, or a camel! The point is to find a way to take a short or longer getaway. To help keep your budget intact, go to your favorite park or beach, toting a picnic basket of favorite foods, for a fun local trip.

Travel can also mean hopping on a plane or train or driving to visit a friend or to see a new city. Whatever may be possible for you! The point is to give yourself a new adventure, distracting you from problem-solving, as you wind down and regroup. You can also create new space for solutions to emerge just by writing out your present challenges on paper. As your words and/or your body start moving, toss out everything that's weighing you down!

3. Ask for help: If you have a support system in place, don't be afraid to ask for help. Get help taking things off your plate, help to prioritize what needs to be done—or get help *period* with whatever's going on with you. There is nothing wrong with having a helper in your lifeboat.

Warning: Pride will always try to stop you from asking for help! See that as a yellow light, and not a red one. Slowly, but surely, get what you need…by going down your list of supportive friends, family, or professionals—and then reach out for the help you need!

"The Healing Partner" Question:

What do you need to do to take care of you?

I Speak...

Secret #2
From the Cover up to the Cure

> *"When we are lying to ourselves,
> it is even easier to lie to others."*
> —PerCilla, "The Healing Partner"

IN the late 1980s, at the tender age of seventeen, I had a December wedding. My first husband (I will call him Blair) was himself only 19. Blair was in the Navy, and I was finishing my last year of high school. And, after six months of dating, I proposed to him and he accepted.

Blair had neither chick nor child, and neither did I. He was up for orders to leave San Diego, CA, where we lived, so we made plans to be married and then to reconnect at his new duty station after my high school graduation.

I will never forget my mother coming into my room hours before the wedding. She was walking down the hallway and passed by my room. She noticed that I was in a daze, sitting at the edge of my bed. I was waiting to head to the church, but also contemplating if we were ready to do this thing called marriage. *I know! At that age, what a shocker!*

My mom came into the room and sat down beside me.

"Are you OK?" she asked. "Are you sure you want to do this?" The truth was that I loved him, but both he and I weren't ready.

We were young adults, both with heavy childhood baggage we had not cleared out. We were in love with the love that was needed to fill the void caused by the heavy baggage. And a lot of my motivation in proposing to him was that I loved him, but I was also fearful of not having him in my life (there goes that fear again!).

In my heart I knew I wasn't ready, but I didn't give myself time to realize that. I didn't take time to get real with my thoughts and doubts and fears. I was thinking so much about the idea of being his wife and moving away from San Diego that I could see no further beyond this.

I was also afraid to change my mind hours before walking down the aisle and, frankly, I wanted to prove to myself and to my mother that it was going to work. As much as she loved Blair, Mom was against my marriage from the beginning, because I was so young. I was three months shy of eighteen; so in her mind there was a high probability that I would run off and get hitched without her permission, and this was the only reason she gave her approval.

If I'd given her an inkling of how I was feeling, she wouldn't have hesitated to shut it down and to create some other random event we could have celebrated that day. Unfortunately, I didn't share my truth; instead, I continued lying to myself, about what I wanted at that very moment, which was more time to love on him without losing him.

So, when my mother asked me if I was sure I wanted to be married, I responded in the most confident way I could. I looked her dead in her eyes and gave her a resounding answer.

"Yes! I'm sure I want to do this." I lied.

I Am Healing - Secret #2

I wasn't sure about anything! Coming from an awesome mother of five, among whom I was the eldest, I had given Mom my fair share of disobedience. I don't know how she got through it, but she always did, continuing to show me love and support. Now, though she was giving me an opportunity to be straight with her, I had lied. *When we are lying to ourselves, it's even easier to lie to others.*

The secret to self-care I want to share with you from this personal life story is about the responsibility we have to *self-assess* for our truth, our own internal truth. This is the place where our growth, our mindfulness, and our intention-making come together in their richest form.

Without being conscious of your own inner truth in any situation, you won't be able to make smart, informed decisions or to take the next steps in complicated circumstances that involve more than just you and your own needs. Blair and I at some point came to the realization that, although we weren't ready when we tied the knot, the love we shared could influence us to only unpack our childhood baggage with one another. We made it to almost ten years and, unfortunately, it didn't work out the way we had hoped in the end.

So, let me ask you: What is the truth you've been denying that's keeping you from evolving? What's keeping you in a state of anger, distrust, passivity, over-controlling, fearfulness, lack of love, chaos, or any other disposition that is hindering your progress?

No matter how you arrived at a hindering disposition, *you* are the solution to getting out of it. Whoever did something wrong to you or *you to them*, matters less than the truth you need to speak and the *you* you need to own in order to experience healing. You have the questions, and you are the answer. Coming full circle in this way (from the cover-up to the cure) is an absolute necessity in the process of self-healing and self-care.

With so much going on around you every single day, it can be easy to allow yourself to be swept up in the moment and lose hold of your truth. To make a situation smoother, for example, you take on the unprogressive energy that ignores parts of yourself that might otherwise complicate things, or you might neglect to ask for what you need. Doing this may keep things calm, not rocking the boat for the moment, but the more you ignore the truth within yourself, the harder it becomes to live a peaceful and honest, illusion-free life. It's like layering on mask after mask in order to cover up the real you. Eventually, the *real you* is forgotten and lost almost entirely.

One reason you may have for doing this is that you don't like something within yourself or you're afraid of the outcome if you speak up. Ignoring a part of yourself does not make it go away; it only shoves that part deeper into your soul. When this happens, it makes some aspect of your life a bit tougher. Remember, there is no part of your inner or outer being that is negative, but there can be negative internal dialogue or false perspectives that keep you from moving forward. Each day brings another opportunity to start better, be better, and live better.

Looking within, doing the inner work, speaking truth, owning and loving what you see within you (good, bad, and ugly) is how you protect your energy. It's time to roll up your sleeves and do the work of self-assessing so that your truth will radiate more brightly—from the inside out!

"The Healing Partner" Work

Affirmation

I speak and receive the truth, and let the truth be my guide.

Acknowledgement

Acknowledge any stress that may derive from having a hard time expressing yourself the way you would like to or from saying things you fear you may regret later. Acknowledge any issues with white lies, and plan to correct them. No matter what color your lie is…it's still *a lie*.

Attunement

Throat Chakra – This energy is located in front of the neck (larynx). Clearing the blockage in the throat chakra will assist with areas of speaking your truth, communication, and the inspiration of unleashing your creativity. Depending on your unique situation, there are healers, exercises, and meditations that can assist with this. Do your research for what fits best for you.

"The Healing Partner" Thoughts:

Below is an exercise you can do to find out if there are some truths you are keeping from yourself.

Take a few minutes to calm your mind by breathing deeply. Take five to ten deep breaths, just setting everything else aside in your life. If worries come to your mind, acknowledge them and just set them aside for now.

When you start to feel a sense of peace, go into your heart of hearts and ask yourself: *In the areas of my life where I am facing challenges, what truths are there that I'm afraid to acknowledge? Is there something I'm hiding from myself?*

This can be a tough question to ask yourself, so keep breathing deeply, exhale, and keep asking yourself the question a number of times. If you notice that you are starting to feel anxious, or want to avoid the subject, that may be a sign that there is something you don't want to acknowledge.

Be gentle with yourself; we are all a work in progress, an unfinished masterpiece. It's OK to make mistakes, to get it wrong, to apologize or ask for forgiveness. Just like it's OK to forgive, let things go, and not to punish others for their mistakes. We are not perfect, but there is a perfection in love and honesty. So, whatever comes up during this exercise, accept what is true, accept yourself for being where you're at *right now,* and acknowledge that change is still possible.

Mahatma Ghandi said, *"Be* the change you want to see, in the world." It sounds so simple, yet putting this in motion can prove challenging at times. As you acknowledge your truths, this step isn't asking you to jump right in and suddenly be a whole new person; it's asking you to take the first small step toward the person that you truly are within—and making no excuses for your current shortcomings.

If you find yourself slipping into old habits of picking up the masks you've worn in the past, remind yourself that you only cheat yourself of quality of life every time you aren't your authentic self. Remind yourself of this as many times as you need to until "living as the real you" becomes a new and daily habit.

"The Healing Partner" Question:

What area in my life am I lying to myself?

"The Healing Partner" Question:

What steps can I take to move toward the truth?

I Do...

Secret #3
Fear the Cycle

"By silence, I hear other men's imperfections, and conceal my own!"

—Zeno of Elea

LOOKING back through my life and memories, I remember when my children were just babies and I used to say, "I can't wait until my kids turn eighteen and are grown." I would imagine how close we would be then. But I can tell you that when my eldest three children got to be that age, it wasn't like that. In fact, I buried my eldest son when he was only twenty-three years old. At that time, I began to wish that I had all those years back to do things differently as a parent. In my deep grief, I analyzed myself critically, dwelling on times when I couldn't seem to make things go right, no matter how I tried.

Now I realize that it wouldn't have changed a thing in the mothering of my children. I was the best parent I could be at that age, based on my experiences, my perception of life, and my general know-how at the time—and he was the best son he could be with his youthful resources, as well.

When my firstborn son, David, died, I was living in Japan. I had a long flight home to Virginia in order to lay him to rest. On the flight home, I did a lot of serious thinking about my life and all the time I had missed with my three eldest children; it was coupled with painful guilt. At the time, my second-eldest son was incarcerated, and my daughter and I weren't connected in the way that I felt a mother and daughter should be connected. I had lost one of my sons, and I was struggling with the two eldest of my five children.

Nonetheless, I still entertained the question, *What would I have done differently?* The biggest thing I would've done was love my children unconditionally. I had put conditions on my love in a way that I judged them when they moved in directions that I did not agree with. I didn't learn how to show love and support through listening regardless of their path until later. So, when they were angry with me, I most certainly wasn't going to be the one to pick up the phone and call, even after six months or so.

I was in a place where my fear of being wrong and my stubbornness didn't want to understand that it was OK to call them and say, "I'm sorry we aren't in agreement right now, but we are going to get through it. I just called to say I love you, regardless."

But why had I acted in ways that communicated the opposite of love in the first place? Seriously speaking, there is no need for me to 'rectally' engineer the answer to this question. What I found interesting in revisiting my past and self-assessing, was that *fear* was deep-rooted in me and had always been a tremendous part of my life. I was always afraid. In addition to that, what was deep-rooted in me was also the common denominator, for my actions.

I Am Healing - Secret #3

Now here I was using the silent treatment as a weapon of coercion. I was using it so that my adult children would be fearful of not having me in their lives, in hopes that they'd want me to speak to them so badly that they would oblige my request to change how they made their decisions at the time. It's one thing when your intentions are to totally cut off a relationship you have no desire to mend. But, as much as I would like to tell you something different, the silent treatment was every bit of mental abuse, since I had no desire to cut my adult children off.

I wasn't the mental abuser while they were young. However, I had become the mental abuser by not speaking to them until they spoke to me as young adults. My trauma was not an excuse I could hide behind for what I had become myself. It was an eye-opener for me to face this truth in the course of my healing and become a better person and a better parent for it.

I had to face the fact that I'd done much hiding. I'd wrapped myself up in stunning confidence and a happy face—anything that looked like the opposite of fear. I hadn't let anyone see me afraid, or see my insecurity and pain, so I'd wrapped it up in something people loved to perceive: a joyful mask. It hid all the anxiety, emotional turmoil, and secrets I didn't want others, even those closest to me, to see—*but who the hell was I really fooling?* Only myself! Once a good girlfriend of mine said something interesting to me.

"PerCilla, as long as I've known you—in elementary, middle school, and high school—you have always been so chipper and so happy." My wrapping was so pretty to her that she never knew how I really felt inside.

Before my journey into self-healing and self-care, I would have agreed with her so graciously. However, because my path was changing as I strived to be more authentic with self, I was able to respond to her kind words with transparency.

"Girl, I was happy on the outside, but on the inside, I was dying. I was going through some real *stuff!*" She was shocked, to say the least.

If you'd met me back then, you might never have imagined there was fear within me, either. The energy of fear is one of the most challenging things to face within yourself, but if you don't face it, it will drive you in powerful ways; either it will give you a reason to do courageous things or give you a reason to do stupid sh*t. So, the great lesson that I want to share with you is that the *cycle of fear* in your life has to stop. I finally came to a place where I was sick and tired of being afraid of being powerless all the time…and using fear and control to hurt others.

Fear Has Torment

When you start to work on overcoming fear in your life, the fears you have to combat may be very different from the ones I've spoken about here. For example, you might realize that fear of failure (or even success) is the underlying reason that you procrastinate on things in life. Or you might see that fear is the underlying reason that you have not pursued the job or career path you truly want for yourself. For some, the fear of not being in control of everyone and everything makes you feel powerless and afraid. So, telling people what, when and where to do what you want may be second nature to you, superseding the fact that it's not your place.

You might be amazed by the way fear exists, the inaction and actions it causes in your life like weight gain, lying about your past, present or future, conceit regarding wealth or education, jealousy, damage to relationships and other unhealthy and unkind behaviors that allow you to hide the true you.

One of my clients, whom I will call *Nina,* was in a very difficult situation in her life because of a period of unemployment she had gone through. She realized she needed to do something to get the ball rolling, so she started doing Uber® grocery deliveries. On her first day of work, she had a car full of deliveries when a torrential thunderstorm struck.

Nina became paralyzed in that situation. She was afraid to go out in that torrential downpour. And yet she was also afraid of the consequences of not completing her deliveries. There are truly dangerous situations out there, but many of our fears actually amount to the irrational fear Nina had of walking through a storm. Luckily, she remembered the breathing exercises I taught her. She did some deep breathing and realized that she just had to *persist*, even though it was not the ideal situation.

The next time she jumped out of a car and into the rain, she had this thought: "Why am I afraid of the rain?" Nina did what she needed to do: to check-in with herself, in order to get back to her true self.

In my own story of returning to Virginia to lay my son to rest, three days after I arrived, I found myself in my room late in the evening, while my daughter was in hers. We were stuck in our own separate worlds, despite the tragedy of my son's passing and our own years of disconnection. As the television watched me, instead of me watching it, I started to remember all the things I had reflected on while I was on the flight from Tokyo. I was afraid to reach out to her, not knowing if she was going to be standoffish or return the love I would offer her. I asked

Spirit to give me the willpower and the words, because I needed her to know I was there for her. I needed her to know that I needed her, too.

As I lay there talking to Spirit, finally I got out of my bed and knocked on my daughter's door to see if she was asleep. She was lying in her bed, doodling on her phone. I lay next to her and asked how she was doing. She said she was doing OK. I went on.

"I am so sorry for everything and anything that I may have done to hurt you in the past," I said. Then I did something that I had not done since she was nineteen years old, I reached over and held my twenty-three year-old daughter as if she were a two year-old. It wasn't just grief talking. I knew that I had to change the cycle of fear I was caught in if I wanted a different future with her, and with everyone I loved.

"The Healing Partner" Work

Affirmation

I do foster personal power in healthy ways. I'm confident and in control of every area in my life, because I am worthy of nothing less.

Acknowledgement

Acknowledge the stress that may be coming from a sense of powerlessness. Acknowledge issues with aggressive tendencies and the fact that you have the ability to do things you may later regret.

Attunement

Solar Plexus – This energy is located two inches above the navel. Clearing the blockage in the Solar Plexus chakra will assist with areas of willpower, misusing power, an obsession with control, and other areas. Depending on your unique situation, there are healers, exercises, and meditations that can assist with this. Do your research for what fits best for you.

"The Healing Partner" Thoughts:

When you start to see how pervasive fear is in your life and how it can affect your excessive need for control of the environment or of people, you might be surprised. It's a frightening world! Fear is something that doesn't just go away. It has to be *managed* daily.

So, I suggest you set aside a dedicated time each and every day to unblock any fear or other compromised energy you are holding onto. By giving yourself five or ten minutes a day to focus on your own needs and your own positive, fluid flow of energy, you open up your inner self for the flow of peace to continue.

Take just five minutes in the morning to check in with yourself. Five minutes of calm can help set the mood for your entire day. Take another five minutes before bedtime to do the same; it will help you rest, relax, and rejuvenate your mind in preparation for sound sleep and peaceful dreams.

Self-care and self-healing aren't always about fixing *everything* right then and there. Sometimes the best self-care you can give yourself is merely the time, space, and permission to feel whatever it is you need to feel. The key to this, however, is to make sure any stuck feelings or thoughts that get released don't take over your consciousness. Let them come up, acknowledge they exist, and then let them flow downstream....

That idea brings us to our next powerful self-care tip. Remember, the better you become at facing your fears, the more *fearless* you will become.

"The Healing Partner" Question:

What fears am I facing?

"The Healing Partner" Question:

What steps can I take to get passed them?

I Love...

Secret #4
When you Forgive, You Live!

"If you don't heal the hurt, you'll bleed all over the people who didn't cut you."
– Unknown

I'VE always admired movies where the female's identity front was that of a mom, a businesswoman, or even a loner with two cats—and in a flash she'd become the "She-ro" that laid at least fifty bandits on their backs before you could shout, "Wait, what the heck just happened?"

I mean brutal, beg-for-mercy, drop-to-your-knees, "I've taken everything, including your dignity, and if you even blink the wrong way…I'll take your last breath"- She-ro's! Yeah, that type of movie! And who, pray tell, is that woman in the back of the theater, yelling "Hell, yeah!" between scenes in a high-pitched voice. Yup! That would be me.

I never sought out the training these feisty Kill Bill actresses (or their stunt doubles) acquired, but trust me: I have imagined myself doing some form of Matrix martial arts download, at least a time or two! Before really delving into my self-healing and self-care, forgiving my abusers was the last thing on my mind, believe me.

On the contrary, I'd thought about kicking their asses and taking names. Heck, with skills like that, I could blow off some steam and dance to the remix of "I Will Survive." But intentionally putting my hands on someone to hurt them physically has never been my thing. While doing my inner work, my *I AM* yearned to forgive freely, instead of holding on to the weight of my anger. Besides that, prison isn't a place I'd ever want to be. So I found other ways to blow off steam. For the record, I did take up boxing, and I loved it; but then, while it is stress relieving, it lacks a full energy clearing.

Overcoming the sexual abuse that I suffered as a young girl has been one of the most significant challenges I've had to face in life. Violation of this nature forever changes a person. For many years it hindered my growth in ways I could not even see at the time; it also expanded my will to survive and to be cautious.

I tried to forgive my father and the woman and other young men who abused me, because that was what the people in church encouraged me to do. They said I had to forgive because God wants me to be forgiving. So, I tried, and while doing so, I was speaking forgiveness out of my mouth, but my energy and heart didn't match what I articulated. The problem was that I was trying to move toward forgiving my abusers because I was encouraged to do so, based on my Christian religion. It wasn't because I was making an effort for the true loving energy and the Spirit within me that wanted and needed to embrace the process in order to get to the place of forgiveness.

I went through a period where I tried to speak about the things I endured with some of my paternal family members. Unfortunately, some of them just kind of swept what had happened under the

I Am Healing - Secret #4

rug or doubted my truth…and some were very supportive. Most of them didn't want me to speak about it or bring it up.

Before her passing, I eventually talked about my abuse with my grandmother, and I asked her why she never sought out help for my father. My grandmother was very supportive and honest with me. She never made me feel like she didn't believe me, and she didn't give me any excuses. She shared her truth with me, and I respected her for that. I'm so grateful that she was open enough to even listen to me—and she was ever-so-careful about being honest and authentic with her answers, instead of telling me what I wanted to hear.

Fact is, when my father came out of my grandmother's womb, he wasn't an abuser. As a tiny child, we show the love that's shown to us, not just by our parents, but by the circle of people in our lives, as well.

My grandmother had a glass eye because she'd lost her left eye at the hands of my grandfather. She told me she literally watched her eyeball fly across the room. That was the kind of dad my father had. When I thought about that I realized that as we all have tough experiences growing up, and in our responses to them, we either *become* what we've experienced, or we fight to become the *opposite* of it. Either way, we are affected.

My father never shared his story with me, but I feel he definitely repeated his father's abusive behavior, and that perhaps in being incarcerated—instead of being helped—his selectively unloving ways and thoughts became even more heightened. It doesn't take a rocket scientist to figure out that our current correctional system is not rehabilitative, so I do believe it kept him in a place where he continued to want to put other people through the same or similar abuse in the most manipulative ways he could. It left him with *selective* or very little compassion and respect, not just for me, but for people in general. *Is this who my father truly was?* No.

Who needs to forgive a being like that? I did.

Why, because I also believe that my father's abusive nature was not the substance of his *I Am*. This brought me to the conclusion that all who had harmed me were people who'd had traumatic experiences they'd never dealt with honestly. Not dealing with their own experiences didn't allow them to show the love, kindness, and compassion needed to respect other peoples' boundaries and personal space. In time, some would come out of denial and get what they needed to get it right, and some would never see the break of day. Instead, they would choose to remain in an energetically blocked, dim, unhealthy place, completing their prison sentences locked inside themselves and/or behind bars for the hurt they had caused others. In my humble opinion, prison is the pathway to half-assed healing or to no desire to heal at all.

Either way, the challenge I now faced was not about *them*. It was about me choosing to take back the power I had surrendered to their demands in my abuse and about finding a way to truly forgive. Unforgiveness was keeping *me* from living the highest and best life I could live. What was super vital for me now came with finding a way to transform the energy that had touched me in dim and cruel ways. Forgiving in *my time* and through a process that I could embrace, without being artificial, just felt right. With the willingness of my *I AM* and the energy work I committed myself to, I made the effort to move forward.

I know some of you who've experienced something similar are wondering how I can even think about forgiveness for such acts. I'm not saying I condone any abuser's selfish and cruel actions. However, I do know that we all need help with and deliverance from our twisted thoughts, and I know that help is available for those who are willing and open to receive it.

There was no excuse for what my abusers did, and I can't change the past and pretend it didn't happen. However, I can take back my power and stop the ripple effect of unforgiveness within myself and toward them. If we're being perfectly honest, we all have our twisted thoughts and ugly faces.

There is a Japanese proverb going around the internet that says this: "The first face, you show to the world. The second face, you show to your close friends, and your family. The third face, you never show anyone. It is the truest reflection of who you are."

We have inner thoughts and these three faces—and some of them are not very pretty; thus, we all need forgiveness from someone.

The Consequence of Unforgiveness

In working with many clients, I have seen that an inability to let go of old pain and hurts can cause a lot of problems, sometimes even physical ailments. When Mara came to see me, she had headaches and back pain. After working with her, it became clear that the pain she was carrying was left over from the fact that her mom had left her at a young age, and never came back. Her father had also died when she was thirteen years old.

Mara had tried to reconnect with her Mom as an adult but had never gotten the mother/daughter relationship she'd wanted. Once she had gone to visit her mother in Houston to try and connect with her.

She knocked on the door of her mom's house and her mother

didn't invite her inside. She just stepped outside onto the porch and talked with her there. It was even raining outside. Can you imagine how badly that hurt Mara?

I did some energy work with Mara, which I will talk more about in Chapter 8, and that helped her let go of the pain she'd carried around her mother's failings. Our session brought some relief to her throbbing headaches, and she was able to let go of the heavy burden she'd carried for years. Letting go of the pain others have caused us can be difficult, but it is essential in the healing process. What was most essential was the willingness and openness Mara had to do the opposite of what she'd been doing, in order to receive the self-healing, she needed.

When I think of my relationship with my father and my other abusers, I'm first grateful for making it through the process of forgiveness to the place where I experienced the willingness to change some long-held feelings, like anger. Having grown up in a period of time where I had access to people who helped me a lot didn't hurt, either.

Thankfully I was open enough to receive that help in the moments when I needed it. I had people in my life that reached out to me in a way that made it possible for me to think about what had happened and not bottle it all up and refuse self-healing. It opened me up to the possibility of trusting life again, which I don't believe my abusers had ever had or had simply resisted or ignored.

So, I chose to forgive them. It took time, but that *choice* was the door to change. And trust me…it changed everything! It helped me to show much more motherly affection to my children and led to my growth in making peace within myself and in several different areas of my life. It led to you reading these words today.

"The Healing Partner" Work

Affirmation

I love, and I am open to giving and receiving love. As I accept and forgive myself, I extend love to others.

Acknowledgement

Acknowledge the stress that may be coming from a disconnection with self and others. Acknowledge the issues that may come from hatred, vengeance, guilt, grief, fear, lack of forgiveness, feeling stuck, and hiding.

Attunement

Heart Chakra– this energy is located in the center of the chest. Clearing the unforgiveness, deep hurt, and other blockages of the heart chakra will assist in bringing relief in this area. Depending on your unique situation, there are healers, exercises, and meditations that can assist with this. Do your research for what fits you best.

"The Healing Partner" Thoughts

Because unforgiveness is an especially challenging form of energy blockage, I want to share a powerful technique that I learned from the teacher, Adyshanti, while watching Oprah on TV! Shout out to Oprah's "Super Soul Sunday"!

◊ Close your eyes and see who and/or what is bothering you.

◊ Now, in your mind's eye, watch it move to a chair across from you.

◊ Say what you need to say to it, and then forgive it.

◊ After you forgive it, bless it, and wish it well.

◊ Still, with your eyes closed, let it go and watch it leave. (I add light healing music to this exercise; so can you if you'd like.)

In most cases, this exercise of forgiveness and letting go will provide you with a sense of closure and release. Sometimes, however, you will reach an element or circumstance that you don't want to forgive or bless, where something keeps you from letting it go. For deep wounds like that one, it will generally take returning to this exercise many times and/or asking for help from your Higher Source and external professional help.

The first time I tried this method, it worked. But the next time I tried it, I got to step three and understood that I hadn't actually let that situation go. So now I use this process to help me better understand the things I'm letting go of and the things I'm bullsh'tting myself with. Many times we think we've let something go, but there can be one little trigger and then all of a sudden we are right back where we started with our unforgiveness.

It's also important to say by no means am I perfect; no one is, and it may take time to truly let go. So, know that it's OK—and that you can work on forgiveness and letting some things go in your own time. As I've said before, no one is chasing you, this is not a race, and *you get to choose* how to distribute and sift through and nurture your energy. Just make sure you're self-encouraging what lies deep within and not just ignoring it!

"The Healing Partner" Question:

Who do you need to forgive -or- Who needs your forgiveness?

"The Healing Partner" Question:

How can you allow that to happen?

I Feel...

Secret #5
The Process of Sifting

> *"The reason why we have two ears
> and only one mouth is that we may
> listen the more and talk the less."*
> – Zeno of Citium

BEING a parent is not always easy. We do the best we can, based on what we know and have at the time. There is no manual for raising little ones, or for when they become grown adults, for that matter.

My children from my first marriage experienced more than they should have in their childhood. Because I wasn't consistent with my own therapy, along with my half-assed self-care, fearfulness had me shielding and overprotecting them in times that really didn't call for it. Despite these and other mistakes I made, my eldest son overcame severe learning disabilities and acquired a full academic college scholarship. My only daughter attended college and was always snazzy in business. She helped manage one of my companies—and a couple of nightclubs for investors. My third child left the United States and opened a small hat company in Japan, where he also picked up paid gigs performing his own music in Japanese hip-hop nightclubs.

Based on all their accomplishments, it's easy to see my kids were very capable of making their own decisions. But for a long time, when a problem came up in their lives, I tried to be their problem solver. When a challenge came up, I got as much information as possible, dissected it all out, thought of all the possible angles on it, and then said to them, "OK, you need to do this, this, and this."

I used all my energy to home in on resources and do what I could and to figure out how to make whatever problem they were venting about better. As most parents do, I sacrificed my own joy and harmony in order to contribute to theirs. I gave them whatever it was I could offer; my time, my money, my tears. *All of it.*

The thing was that my contribution wasn't always received in a grateful way. Mostly because they didn't want me involved—or didn't tell me the whole story for fear of my disappointment. But I'd insert myself, without waiting to be asked for my help. *Why?* Because I thought I knew what was best for them.

My children made some great decisions and some wrong ones. Some of my kids were incarcerated for reasons both warranted and unwarranted. A judge gave my nineteen-year-old son—fresh out of college and with no priors—a felony charge and 5+ years of prison time for spray painting gang graffiti on a wall. *Had I taught him better?* Absolutely! *Did he deserve that insanely excessive sentence?* Hell, no! But we both had to live with his mistake. Thank God, most of it was suspended.

When he did his jail time, I was doing jail time too—mentally, that is. How I prayed that nothing would happen to him while he was away! Where I went wrong was that at the time, I thought we both had to figure out what was going to be best for his life, but actually that was not my job.

For a long time, I carried guilt for my childrens' wrong decisions that had cost them time behind bars. Thinking I wasn't a good mother, I worried about what people would say about me, based on my children's wrong decisions. Of course, from a bigger perspective, I can't truly call them wrong decisions. Sometimes we go in what seems like the wrong direction until it leads to finding the right direction.

The most painful lesson for me was coming to accept that I don't have the final say on how my grown children choose to live their lives. Regardless of all the nights I cried for them, stayed up late trying to figure out how to help them out of a situation, and/or lay awake trying to figure out how to change their minds if they didn't like my solution for them, each of them showed me that they had to make their *own* choices and implement their own solutions. I could no longer conduct their symphonies. I had to let them experience their own pain, go through their own mishaps, learn their own truths, and find their own joy and harmony.

I did finally learn this lesson, however. I realized that a lot of what I was doing was actually hurting them, and me. It prevented them from seeing the decisions they made that were self-destructive. And some of the answers I gave weren't always right *for them also.* When I ran to the scene and "saved" them, they never learned the tough lessons of life, and neither did I.

When it hit me that this was true, I was like: *Wait a minute! I'm feeling a whole lot of pain here, and this is not my shit. I'm carrying a load that no one asked me to carry. And it's not serving me, or them. So why am*

I holding on to it?

Yes, we're the parents and I get that. But that's when I realized that the way I can truly be the best help to them is to let go of *their* load and let them figure it out. That also gave me back the energy I needed to carry and deal with my own. As much as I loved them, I couldn't live both my life and theirs, too. I was trying to make them follow my recipe for life, rather than allow them to follow their own. My plan was to be the head chef. But in reality, I had been invited to *their* dinner table, and I wasn't being grateful for my role as the guest.

This point of understanding surfaced for me when I finally became grateful that they even *wanted* to share what they were going through with their mother; that they wanted to share their lives with me. Appreciating this fact put me in a better place to just *listen* to my children, and not *fix* everything for them. I may or may not like what I was hearing, but having me as a listener was what they each really needed in their process of learning the lessons of life.

Sift It, and Let It Go!

Now, you may or may not have children, and if you do you may not have the exact same parental challenges that I faced. But I think the lesson here that we can all learn from is that we need to take time to *sift through* life, asking ourselves if there are behaviors, we have that are counter-productive—and *eliminate* them!

Have you adopted an approach to life, or relationships, or people that is creating more difficulties than necessary? The reason I've shared this example from my life with my children is that, it's so powerful. Amazingly, the thing that you might be doing in offering to help may not be helping you *or* the people around you. It might be your habit of hindrance or your habit of enabling! It was for me.

Sifting through your life and asking this question about your way of being with other people or your way of approaching different challenges can sound like a monumental task—one that seems tedious and maybe even terrifying. But if you breathe deeply and reflect more completely on this idea, you will recognize that there are tremendously valuable insights in the pile of possibilities that your life has collected thus far. If you are willing to commit yourself to doing this deep self-inventory, you will undoubtedly recognize what is important for you to focus on—and what is important to let go of. Your *I AM* will provide you with the energy needed to focus on the sifting process of self-healing and self-care.

The process of separating, seeking, and *letting go of* is actually ongoing and unending. But if you remind yourself of the truth that no one is chasing you, and it isn't a race or a competition, you will find yourself mastering the art of knowing what to discard and what to hold on to; of knowing what does and does not serve you well.

Toxic thoughts about yourself, negative comments of others, unproductive work habits, and unhealthy choices on what to fill your mind, body, and spirit with can fill your soul with waste matter and prevent you from uncovering your greatness and happiness. If you have been accustomed to those habits, choices, and ways of being for many years, it can be extremely difficult to let go of them. Although they poison your soul, they may be the only things you know. They have a feeling of familiarity that is easy to confuse with comfort. How can you free up space for newness and flowing energy in your experience of life? One by one, you must release each of the toxic thoughts and the cruel comments of others. You must let go of the same negativity that you give and the self-doubt that fills your soul. This will make room inside yourself for positive self-talk, moments of reflection, and uncovering your highest and best intentions. This active intention releases the free-flowing, positive, and balanced energy of a healthy life…gracefully moving you forward!

While it didn't happen overnight, I've finally arrived at the understanding that if other people aren't kind, empowering, and willing to offer good intentions, it's OK not to give a damn about what those people think anymore—and it's none of my business what they think, anyway!

This awareness and new positive vision for my life has been so freeing. And to get there, I had to discover that what *we* think about ourselves is the only thing relevant. The energy in our thinking radiates and creates a ripple effect. In my case, I had to intentionally and purposefully focus on not feeling guilty for mistakes my kids had made or the ones I'd made as a parent, in order to arrive at this new place of understanding.

I want to encourage you to replace your toxic self-thoughts with empowering and positive ones. Replace your poor work habits with ones that allow you to grow and evolve within yourself and advance the process of coming back to your *I AM*. Choose to shift your mind, body, and spirit choices from unhealthy and damaging ones to transcendent and enlightening ones. You can choose to do this. You have that power. You have that agency. Your energy is yours. It always has been…no matter how life or circumstances have made you feel.

Once you let go of all the things that aren't really serving you well, and you take the time to see what you can learn for your own self, you will experience tremendous growth as a human being. You will also empower others.

In my own situation with my children, I realized that I had to stop taking on their pain, worry, and doubt. The work is up to them. That decision wasn't easy. Once I made it, I went through a period of time where I beat myself up over it. I kept thinking: *If I'm not doing it, who's going to help them?* I was literally beating myself up because I wasn't making their decisions, instead of celebrating the fact that I was getting back to my own joy by not carrying their load, one they were fully capable of carrying, one that made them stronger to carry themselves.

I had to remember that I wasn't put on this earth to *fix* anybody. I was put on this earth to *be*. To be in existence and to be in love. That's it. My job is not to fix my kids. My job is not to fix my friends or my siblings. My job is to exist in love. My job is to put *me* in the best space so that I can vibrate at the highest and best energy level possible—and for me to just be.

"The Healing Partner" Work

Affirmation

I feel joy in living freely and abundantly. I give joy while living in my freedom, to accept others and new experiences.

Acknowledgement

Acknowledge the stress you may have from unhealthy interactions or relationships, lack of a sense of your life's importance, and your need to learn how to use emotion to connect with others without losing your identity.

Attunement

Sacral Chakra –This energy is located two inches below the naval. Clearing the blockages connected to a lack of discovering the enjoyment of life in order to create deeper, more loving relationships will assist in bringing relief to this chakra. Depending on your unique situation, there are healers, exercises, and meditations that can assist with this. Do your research on what fits best for you.

"The Healing Partner" Thoughts:

Maybe you're asking, "How do I know which thoughts, feelings, and energies no longer serve me?"

A good place to start is with the thoughts you have that are troubling you. When you find yourself upset about something, you can ask yourself if the way you are thinking about that thing will bring you any answers. Ask if it's bringing you closer to the positive results you'd like to see in your life. If the answer is *no* to either of those questions, it may be a toxic thought or feeling, and you may need to let it go.

The same question can be asked about your work habits, how you handle your relationships, and the choices you make for mind, body, and spirit. As you examine the issues in your life that are bothering you, first ask yourself, *Is this really my business, or is this someone else's business?* If it's someone else's business, then let go of it. We're not here to fix anyone but ourselves.

If you find that it *is* your own issue that you need to resolve, then take the time you need for self-care. If you simply continue to ask yourself and your Higher Source what's preventing you from emanating love, and then listen quietly, you will be amazed at the wisdom that comes to you. So many good answers come to us in silence.

"The Healing Partner" Question:

What in my life is no longer serving me?

I Know...

Secret #6
Forward, Growing, Evolving!

> *"Self-care and self-healing should be
> in the state where optimism and action
> are continuous and unceasing; going on forever.
> That's how the evolution of ourselves can happen."*
> – PerCilla, "The Healing Partner"

WHEN I think about forward momentum, I think about my mother. There should be a picture in the dictionary of a short, black woman approximately 5'5" tall, with a sassy, short haircut right next to the word momentum! When I say my mother (Ms. Jacquie) is the epitome of it, I don't just mean "take the bull by the horns and go for it" momentum. I mean "take the bull by the horns, marinate it, and fillet that sucker!"

Ms. Jacquie moved forward even when she was straight-up terrified of the consequences she could face for doing so. When I was eight years-old my mother fled from the East Coast to the West Coast to hide from my abusive father. She had very little money—just the small amount my father's mother secretly gave her. They had devised a plan that she could flee with her three smallest babies and send for the last two when she got there. My grandmother and mother both knew what my father was capable of, and both were afraid of what would become of my mother if she stayed in the area.

Mom wasted no time when she got to California. She procured enough resources from social services and family to get my sister and me to the West Coast as soon as she could. Working hard and acting fast to create a better life for us was not only challenging, but also nerve-wracking, because Mom had to do it while hiding from my father. We stayed with a family member at first, and then with a family friend. Within few weeks of Ms. Jacquie's arrival, she had a job, a two-bedroom apartment in southeast San Diego, and government assistance to help feed us.

My Father eventually found my mother and caused brutal injuries to her head and body that resulted in her spending days at the hospital in a coma. However, even that didn't stop her. Ms. Jacquie was always thinking ahead, thinking about the safety of her five kids, as well as herself. She was so ahead of the game that somehow during her hospital stay, her divorce attorney and his wife took us into their home so that social services wouldn't separate us. I have no idea how Mom and the attorney pulled that off, knowing all the red tape she would have had to go through for something like that to happen.

Mom was always putting plan A, B, and C into action when it came to what she wanted in life. So, once she made her mind up, it was pretty much a wrap; she never let anything get in the way of seeking that better life.

One year after getting back on her feet, Mom started going to night school. She kept at it until she graduated from San Diego Community

I Am Healing – Secret #6

College. She was selected for a scholastic achievement award and was listed on the National Dean's List. I will never forget the day my mother graduated with honors, with all five of her kids in the audience cheering her on. Ms. Jacquie now held two degrees, one in criminal justice and one in psychology—and she didn't stop there; she became a published poet. Later on, when all her kids moved out, she went on to help other parents as an instructor for the positive parenting programs within the court system, and as a court-appointed special advocate for neglected and abused children.

To say that my mother leaped over hurdles in life is an understatement. And the entire time she studied and supported us all, she *still* had to be a mom taking care of five children. She endured nights of not eating so that *we* could eat. She even survived raising us through our teen years as a single parent, which was at times extremely difficult for her.

Before remarrying, my mom had no husband to console her and no mother to consult, but she did have some "lifeboat" friends and family members and healing partners such as pastors and peer support that she could turn to occasionally. And let me be clear, without fail she always turned to her Higher Power, her Source, for help.

My mom found ways to do self-care, even when she couldn't afford to do so. Somehow, she found a way to bring joyful energy to herself and to her family members.

Some of those times were when we'd sit together, balling and twisting up week-old *San Diego Union-Tribune* newspapers to throw into the fireplace (yup…sometimes we couldn't even afford firewood).

Believe me, we were excited about it. Knowing this occasional gathering would lead to either dancing to tunes like Bill Withers

"Lovely Day" or Diana Ross' "I'm Coming Out," we were content. It didn't even matter if it came down to just sitting together, watching the fire. We were truly content. Even as I think about it now, for me it was better than a trip to Disneyland. We were together, loved, and we had each other, just the way Ms. Jacquie wanted it to be.

I'm sure Mom must have also faced so many other challenges she never shared. But nothing came between her mindset of perpetual motion in her mind, body, and spirit. It's what she taught all her kids, whether we chose to receive the lesson, or not. I'm not saying Ms. Jacquie was perfect, but she set the bar damn high as a mom who recovered from some pretty severe life challenges…and kept moving forward.

In one way or another we are all recovering from and coping with human life experiences. Some of us are also recovering from violence, abandonment, substance abuse/alcoholism, mental health disorders, and other forms of trauma. Or we may suffer deprivation in the physical, emotional, cultural, spiritual, or the educational sense. These trying circumstances can each present obstacles and stumbling blocks that can keep us stuck. This is precisely why self-healing and self-care is necessary and can help us develop the resilience it takes to stay on the pathway, moving forward. If you're wondering the difference between self-healing and self-care, know that self-healing guarantees our continuous momentum and self-care puts the practice in place.

Optimism and Action= Growth

Throughout our journey together thus far we've discussed the idea of *growth* in many different ways. The thought I want to share here, is that forward momentum means a commitment to always strive with everything you have to build the life you want for yourself. It's a profoundly personal experience and decision, one that I hope this book has empowered you to embrace in the healthiest way. Let nothing keep you from the best life you can live. Nurture yourself into being entirely self-loving, continuously self-healing, and comfortable in your own body, while advancing your self-worth and practicing intentional self-care.

The point of the story is that the ideas I've shared about self-care and self-healing should be in the state where optimism and action are continuous and unceasing; going on forever. That's how the evolution of ourselves *can* be, if we choose to evolve. I'm not saying anyone should be a workaholic; remember; we're speaking of healing and care!

Also, keep in mind that the motion we've referred to in these pages is both external and internal. That means that even if your body is sitting still, your mind and spirit can be moving forward. The point of forward momentum from a self-healing and self-care standpoint is that you are always doing something to work toward a better life, a more contented soul, and a more peaceful existence.

At times forward momentum will seem exhausting, but with the right tools, mindset, options, and a great guide/healing partner, you can learn to move forward at your own pace, always growing and evolving. Your goals are attainable, and you hold the power, right now, to move a little bit closer to achieving them. Change your potential energy into taking one healthy action. You'll get the ball rolling and start the forward momentum!

"The Healing Partner" Work

Affirmation

"I know of the harmony, wholeness, and oneness within me."

Acknowledgement

Acknowledge the stress from feeling unaided and disconnected from your Higher Source or Higher Self, whatever that represents for you.

Attune

Crown Chakra–This energy is located at the top and center of the head. Clearing the blockages connected to the lack of spiritual progression or lack of purpose will assist in bringing relief to this chakra. Depending on your unique situation there are healers, exercises, and meditations that can assist with this. Do your research for what fits *you* best.

"The Healing Partner" Thoughts

Throughout these pages I've offered ways to handle many of the challenges on this pathway through life and warned you of the negative self-talk that can impede your progress. This lesson is all about keeping your self-healing work in motion, recognizing that when moving forward is more difficult than usual, it may be a signal that you need to address some self-care need and set yourself up with the resources necessary to ensure your continued progress.

My exercise for you here is to make a "Self-Care Plan." You don't need a long, complicated plan to begin with, just some simple goals. You need a picture or description of the person you want to be and the life you want to have. Start with one page, a paragraph, or even just one sentence. It's OK to not get it right the first time. Keep going. If you're more visual, create a vision board for yourself to illustrate what you are moving toward.

Every attempt to move forward is one more step toward the truth. Remind yourself that it's OK to fail. This will help you accept failure in the moment and *move on* without regrets or negative self-talk.

A small action plan can be as simple as planning to wake up by a certain time each day. It can be as complicated as planning the entire day out, hour by hour. It can even be making a commitment to make your bed every morning!

Just be sure you don't over-plan and that you're ready to make changes in the plan on the fly. We want forward motion, but we don't want to add more stress to your life in the process. Do what feels right, comfortable, and attainable. Also, check out the book *The 5 Second Rule*, by Mel Robbins. It also will inspire you to make small action plans that keep you in forward momentum.

"The Healing Partner" Question:

Choose the area(s) in your life where you want to grow more financially and/or physically?

_____
_____
_____
_____
_____
_____
_____
_____
_____
_____
_____
_____
_____
_____
_____
_____
_____
_____
_____
_____
_____
_____
_____
_____

"The Healing Partner" Question:

Choose the area(s) in your life where you want to grow more emotionally and/or spiritually?

_____
_____
_____
_____
_____
_____
_____
_____
_____
_____
_____
_____
_____
_____
_____
_____
_____
_____
_____
_____

"The Healing Partner" Question:

Write (1) thing to start your plan toward growth and add names of (2) two peers who you believe will morally support you to reach those goals?

_____
_____
_____
_____
_____
_____
_____
_____
_____
_____
_____
_____
_____
_____
_____
_____
_____
_____
_____
_____
_____
_____
_____
_____
_____

I See...

Secret #7
Make the Most of Missteps and Mistakes

*"The point is, you didn't fail:
You learned what not to do next time."*
– PerCilla, "The Healing Partner"

IT was my father who taught me how to ride a bike. As you can imagine from what I've shared about him, it wasn't a picture-perfect, made-for-television teaching moment with my father, but at least he did take the time to hold the handlebars to steady me and slowly instructed me on the proper way to stay balanced on the bike. Then he went back, sat on the porch, and shouted a few more directions at me.

I put my foot to the pedal and nervously took off. Within moments, of course, I lost my balance and fell to the ground. As I lay there crying, he didn't come running to help me up or to offer me any comfort and encouragement. He merely sat there, watching me. After a minute or two, he called out to me.

"Now get up, dust yourself off, and try it again!"

The words he shouted that day have stuck with me my whole life, and for that I am grateful. For a long time they simmered within me, along with my resentment that they weren't spoken in a more loving way. *Should he have come over to comfort me, help me to my feet, and wipe my tears away? Probably.* His response was definitely not ideal parenting.

After a lot of healing over the years, however, I came to see that in that moment my father was giving me the best he was capable of giving. For that reason, I understand today that his words of *tough love* can be motivational for me, if I let them be. And he was right: I most certainly couldn't learn to ride my bicycle from the ground floor position. The ground may have caught my fall, but it was not serving the purpose I set out on. If I was going to learn to ride the bike, I had to do exactly as he said.

Hopefully these words will serve to motivate you, as well: When you fall or fail at something the first time, remember these words, let them resonate within you, and take action. *Get up, dust off, and try again!*

Often we do not get to decide how the experiences of life will come to us or play out, but we are always able to choose our *response* to circumstances. And I've seen where our choices in how we respond to difficult situations are absolutely tied to our self-healing and self-care.

I'm sure you've seen the kinds of people who seem to breeze through difficult experiences without a scratch. Know that we all get *something* from our experiences, even if it's only a memory that becomes a future teachable moment. Then, there are some who come out the other side of a difficult time feeling beaten, bruised, and maybe even defeated—never seeming to be able to get back on the bike at all. *So, how can we become like the first kind of person? What does it really mean* to get up, dust off, and be ready to try again with a fresh mind, a brighter outlook, and an open heart?

Falling Is Not Failing—If We *Learn* From It

How can you make the most of a misstep in life? Though I hated the lesson at the time, returning to this three-step model for making the most of mistakes has been very helpful to me.

◊ Get Up. Getting up is recognizing that you are the ultimate guardian of your own well-being. When your circumstances or experiences knock you off that bicycle you've been trying so hard to learn—even when others around you are not supporting you to the extent you know you need—recall this first step, muster your strength out of love for your life and what you want, and *get the hell up!*

◊ Dust yourself off. Dusting yourself off is forgiving yourself and letting go of the things that do not serve you well, which puts you in a better position to move on. Earlier, I mentioned *The 5 Second Rule* by Mel Robbins. Robbins says, "Knowing what to do will never be enough." Next, you actually have to do it!

◊ Try Again. Trying Again is going after the life that you want for yourself again, and again, and again, until you get it, or until you change your mind and do something else. You're not good at tennis? OK, play chess, or get your tail back out on that tennis court and practice until you get better at it, if what you want to be is a tennis player!

Falling Is Never Graceful

There are lots of reasons we "fall off the bike" in life. We fall from the remnants of our experiences with an abusive parent or in a dysfunctional household, an unhealthy and unsatisfying relationship, our own parenting mistakes, incarceration, failed fitness goals, not meeting school or career goals, poor health, family division, overdrawn bank account, homelessness, joblessness, or even the death of someone we love. Some of these were, possibly, events you were a part of, but they are not who you are.

Falling is painful on many levels. It can cause us to doubt ourselves and our abilities. We can doubt that we even deserve the things we want, at all. Who says this is true? Who's business is it?

After we have fallen, the disappointment in ourselves or others can keep us focused in the wrong direction: backwards. Then, instead of jumping back on the bike, we shuffle along a dim path, look behind ourselves instead of ahead of ourselves, and hold our breath, afraid to try again.

We're gripped with the memory of failure, reliving it over and over again in our heads, beating ourselves up with our words, and/or placing blame. Please stop with the negative self-talk and blame; it won't help you at all. I've been on this track and I had to "piss or get off the pot" to get going in the right direction again!

The secret to learning how to do this is to become acutely aware of how you speak to yourself inwardly. Begin to notice and stay mindful of the tone your inner monologue takes. Would you talk to someone you love in the same way you are speaking to yourself? If not, know that it is urgent to your self-healing that you let that negative self-talk go. Peace, comfort, and kindness are your goal, not that self-loathing and down-talk you may have gotten in the habit of speaking.

Taking responsibility for how you want to move forward and making room for kindness to yourself is an absolute necessity of growth. Doing so will help you be grateful for whatever comes out of your experience of "falling off the bike" in life. It will help you see that everything is a learning opportunity, a way to grow and change and learn what hasn't worked for you. So, are you *bitter*, or *better*?

How do we gain resilience, which is the all-important first element in self-care and self-healing? First of all, by just accepting that sometimes we fall short of our expectations; that's understood. And sometimes it's a big fall! But if we get back to the three steps previously mentioned, our fall can become a learning experience, rather than a catastrophe. This takes a shift in perspective, but it's well-worth the effort to shift it. The point is, you didn't fail; you learned what *not* to do next time. So, if it doesn't pan out to reach your goal the first time (or even the fifth), remember: get up, dust off, and try again!

"The Healing Partner" Work

Affirmation

I see beyond my physical self and trust my intuition.

Acknowledgment

Acknowledge the stress from not being able to trust what's coming next in your life, or from being unable to see the bigger picture in front of you.

Attunement

Brow Chakra–This energy is located between the eyebrows. Clearing the blockage in the Brow chakra will assist in the ability to see more than what is in front of us or see more than where we are at the moment. Depending on your unique situation there are healers, exercises, and meditations that can assist with this. Do your research for what fits you best—and pursue it!

"The Healing Partner" Thoughts:

Included below are some simple steps to help shift your thinking after a fall, and to get you moving in the right direction on the pathway to a brighter future.

◊ Accept that failure happens to everyone. The failure is not *you*, and you are not the failure. It is not a reflection of your value as a person. It's part of being alive. You've been doing it since you were born: falling, and getting back up. You didn't just learn to walk; you took that first step. This is how you learn.

◊ Failure is a small moment in your life, and it will pass. So, don't allow a failure to define the person you'll become. On the contrary, strive toward becoming the person whose victories outweigh their failure. Once you can accept that "disappointment will happen at times, and when it does, it's a normal part of being," you'll begin to see positive changes.

◊ Permit yourself to feel disappointed. While failing and making mistakes is natural and normal, it doesn't mean that you won't still feel bad when you fall from your own expectations. It's OK to acknowledge your feelings of disappointment, or even regret. Please don't try to hide them or push them down. Problems crop up when you allow yourself to get stuck in the muck of your disappointment. Acknowledge those feelings…and get back to those three steps!

◊ Reject your distorted sense of self-worth when you fall short of your expectations. Failures and mistakes can cause even the most talented and skilled people in the world to question their worth. It's easy to start viewing yourself as *lesser* than others, but that's not the truth. Reject those views and focus on all you have accomplished so far. One mistake doesn't negate any of the great things you've already done. If you've said or done something kind for someone, start with that.

◊ Write down a list of your most proud achievements and post that somewhere you can see it every day. This subtle reminder will help bathe your mind and spirit in the true you—the one who succeeds because they never give up!

◊ Ask for help. It is always OK to seek help and guidance from a supportive friend, healing partner, a counselor, a community health worker/certified peer recovery specialist, a religious figure or the person you're most comfortable with to help and not judge you. These people can help you develop a healthy sense of pride about your great qualities and your proud moments. They are wonderful resources for helping you take care of yourself.

◊ Be honest with yourself. If your failure was due to a mistake you made, acknowledge what went wrong and find ways to *be* better or *do* better. If the failure wasn't your fault, accept that it was out of your control. Either way, when you review the situation in a nonjudgmental way, by looking inward at only the facts and not the distorted past, you can see the case more clearly and with new eyes, and then move forward.

◊ Accept that it's not personal. History is full of people who've failed repeatedly and then found meaningful success. *How will you know when you've succeeded?* It's different for everyone, but for me, joy is

I Am Healing - Secret #7

the best measure of success.

Hopefully you understand by now that mistakes happen and that "falling below our expectations at times" is a part of life and the evolution of ourselves. Learning to pick ourselves up, dust ourselves off, and try again can be tough, but it's one of the biggest lessons here and can help in every facet of your life: in every relationship, and in every moment of your day.

Resilience and perseverance always triumph. Despite the tools you put in place to help you experience the ride of your life, *if it doesn't work for you, should you give up?* Absolutely Not! There are so many other things you can try while you learn which self-care techniques work best for you. So, get up, dust off, and try again!

"The Healing Partner" Question:

Choose the area(s) in your life where you can grow more financially, emotionally, physically or spiritually?

_____
_____
_____
_____
_____
_____
_____
_____
_____
_____
_____
_____
_____
_____
_____
_____
_____
_____
_____
_____
_____
_____
_____

"The Healing Partner" Question:

What's your plan or the names of (5) five peers who want to help get you there?

_____
_____
_____
_____
_____
_____
_____
_____
_____
_____
_____
_____
_____
_____
_____
_____
_____
_____
_____
_____

Namaste...

The Energy that Flows from Within: Your Chakra Doors

> *"Accepting things we do not understand, means we have to seek first to understand!"*
> —Unknown

I wish I could say I found energy medicine, but it actually found me. It was almost a year after my son passed. A few months after my weight loss surgery, I went on the YouTube® website looking for something else and I came across this chanting music by a woman named Deva Premal. Since the lyrics were in another language, I didn't understand any of the words, but the music was so beautiful that I played it over and over. It calmed me; it soothed my core and resonated with me just a bit deeper than the other inspirational music I played on Sunday mornings.

I began learning the words to Deva's song, listening to them to the point that even my kids started grooving to them, too, as we rode around together in the car. It was remarkable how this one song in particular really spoke to me, though I didn't even know what the words meant. It was called "Tumare Darshan." Then one day I seemed to sense a Voice rise up from within me, giving me a subtle directive.

"Look up the words. See what these words mean." Now, I have heard that quiet inner voice from time to time in the past, but this was different. This loving voice was quieter and more still, with much more clarity. I looked up the words to the song and they resonated with me so deeply that I got goose bumps. Those words were meant for me! I realized that it was not me singing the song—it was a song Spirit was singing to me:

"The season has arrived where I will finally see you and dance with you. With the breathing in of joy, it is time to live in bliss."

The moment I read these words I had the most powerful feeling that this was now *my time* to move to a different level of life. I would no longer live life from a low to medium vibrational energy, but would live a life of oneness, a life of joy and peace that I had never truly known. It seemed as if the words instantly realigned me to a path that I had detoured from, and now was drawn back toward. Only, this path had new developments.

Through the words of a song, the Voice (Spirit) had brought me to a place of inner joy and consistent peace. After reading the meaning of the words, I felt like there was a reintroduction of two deeply close friends that had lost one another and found each other again through song.

"Tumare Darshan" had brought me inner joy with consistency for weeks, and I hadn't even realized it until I heard the Voice of Spirit. I decided that from that point on I would follow Spirit's guidance.

Sometime after that I moved back to Virginia. I was already on my journey of daily meditation, using various guided meditation tools. My kids and husband started noticing I was different. My mother started

I Am Healing – Secret #7

noticing I was different, and other family and friends close to me started noticing the difference in me, also.

Every day was a normal day, and when Spirit shared information, I gratefully accepted it and followed up to see what gifts it would bring. Then one day Spirit told me to look up *energy medicine*. I had never heard the term before, but I typed it into the internet browser and this program popped up at the top of the Google™ list. I was still in amazement that this guiding Voice was actually on point.

What were the odds that such a thing would even exist, since the first time I was hearing it was right at that very moment? With my interest now piqued, I'm thinking, *This freaking place will be in Timbuktu.* I grabbed my cell phone and called the listed number. A lady answered, and I spoke.

"I'm kind of in a small town called Suffolk, Virginia. Can you tell me where the closest energy medicine instructor to me might be?"

"Ma'am," she said, "I believe we have an instructor in Suffolk." I was thinking, *What in the world!* This is so weird and so freaking incredible! I grabbed some scratch paper and, after taking the number down, quickly called the instructor. She invited me for a free session at her home office. The instructor was literally five or ten minutes from my home. *Talk about divine intervention.*

My husband had much doubt but tried not to show it. On the day I arrived for my first appointment, I walked through this lady's house, and I didn't know what to expect. In her sunroom, after an hour or more of conversing and getting to know her and about her energy medicine practice, I was excited to experience the session and talk about the class. She answered all my questions, made me feel safe and comfortable, and invited me to the massage table for a healing touch therapy session.

After she laid me on the table, tucking blankets to cover me, I remember her placing her hands on my ankles and feet. After that, I literally fell asleep. I remember my son's spirit coming and saying some things, but it's very vague. When I woke up thirty to forty minutes later, I felt lighter. I signed up for her next class and I gave her a big hug and, not wanting to take up too much more of her time, I dashed out the door.

I got in my car and, as I put the keys in the ignition, I didn't turn the key because I felt like it wasn't time for me to leave. So, I sat there in a bit of a daze. It was like I was waiting for something, and then it came: the release, the letting go of the rest of the heaviness I was carrying in my human energy field was being freed from my mind, body, and spirit through my tears. I cried for a good thirty minutes, with my vehicle still sitting in front of her house.

After that, I can't tell you *how* I knew but I knew my new journey was *energy medicine*. As I became more aligned…and with each training, another gift emerged. Now, as I am helping others facilitate self-healing in-person, or with distance healing, I often receive information from Spirit, either audibly and/or physically. At times I physically feel what is compromised in a client's body.

Self-Healing Dis-Ease: For Real?

I remember my first time going to class, thinking, I'll be the only one in the room, clueless, trying to feel the human energy field shouting, "Hey! I don't feel anything!" And now here I am helping clients in ways I could have never imagined.

During that first experience in class, I put my hands over this woman's knees. I could feel her energy, but I also heard Spirit directing me to notice that, "Something's going on with her right knee." I asked her about it.

"I just had surgery on that knee two months ago," she said, "but it's still giving me problems."

When that happened, I was like, What!? This really works?! Oh, my gosh! Then fear kicked in. "What if I tell one of my good girlfriends from around the way about this?" I can hear them now: "Girl, please! Whatever you're drinking over there, I'll have two shots and some lotto numbers!"

But seriously, at first (I have to admit it) I was just as amazed and unconvinced as you may be right now. Receiving the healing and facilitating it was two totally different experiences. In all honesty, for a long time I would never have considered any type of alternative medicine like this. Mostly because, I always felt like if it didn't fit in my little box of religious rituals as a Christian, then it could be nothing more than a bunch of hocus pocus. One of the biggest things I realized through this gift of guidance that was given to me, was that Source was so much bigger than the box I had for it.

We all reject things we don't understand. So, I know there are those small few who will think, "Oh she is batshit crazy!" Or even those select few that will try to condemn me to the pit of Hell for practicing energy medicine.

But then, Source would send a beautiful being, one who was so *stuck* and full of pain, so comprehensively tired of the heaviness they have been carrying from their ailments, from their life experiences, or from their physical discomforts that they'd shut out the negative noise, like I do, so that the work of self-healing can be done.

Healing the Healers

When Alice came to me for treatment, she had been a registered nurse for twelve years. She had symptoms of dizziness, nausea, headaches, and insomnia. Her monthly cycle would stay on for ten days, and then go off for seven days. She told me she was only getting one-and-a-half-to- two hours of sleep at night. This went on for months! She also said her hands felt like they were being stuck in electrical sockets. She went to the doctor, and they couldn't find anything wrong with her. They did blood testing and didn't know what it was. She felt like she was dying.

A naturopathic doctor figured out that her adrenal system was shutting down—so much so that it could have been fatal if they hadn't caught it very soon. He put her on a treatment plan, which worked for some time, but after a while all the symptoms started coming back.

Alice was a skeptic when she came to see me, but she came because as a nurse she'd seen people who were at death's door try energy medicine, get better, and walk out of the hospital well. These were people whose doctors thought they were on their way to the morgue! Alice was a believer in science, but she also knew every situation varies. I was so thrilled to learn that after my session with Alice she went home that night and slept for nine hours. She called it "drool on the pillow" sleep! After that, beyond being cured of insomnia, all of her other symptoms went away, also. Her monthly cycle regulated itself, and her cortisol and adrenaline levels went back to normal.

Those of us who neglected self-care for years may find a build-up of blocked energy in our bodies, just as Alice did. What happens is that when energy gets stuck, it becomes heavier and more pressing. It causes symptoms like physical *dis-ease,* or pain. When energy gets stuck,

I Am Healing - Secret #7

it can manifest as depression, anxiety, fatigue, burnout, headaches, insomnia, discomfort, etc. By using your intentions in a heart-centered way, however, with the right training you can facilitate someone else's self-healing, or you can restore your body's damaged energy flow for yourself.

After previously experiencing lots of trauma, stress, and loss in my life, this practice became a priority in my own self-healing process. Practicing wellness is a daily progression. And just like doctors have to see doctors for care, healers have to see healers, also. I wanted to learn more, and eventually I became certified in energy medicine.

As I move beyond my four (of five) certifications as a Healing Touch Practitioner-Apprentice (HTP-A) and into my fifth and final certification as a Healing Touch Practitioner (HTP) (which I'm currently in the middle of completing), energy medicine is part of the work I do with clients daily. I use Healing Touch to help people release the energy that doesn't serve their highest purpose. Without getting all scientific on you… in physics we know that all matter has a field of energy with unmatched frequencies. Getting an MRI and CT done can show this same information. Healing Touch uses the gift of touch to influence the human energy system, specifically the energy field that surrounds the body, and the energy centers that control the flow from the energy field to the physical body. In my opinion, anyone can be a healer, with the right training. Healers have been an instrument for helping a number of clients move energy that has been stuck in painful physical and emotional ways.

It truly is a self-healing therapy, initiated by healers who are only the facilitators/conduits trained on the healing process. The most important thing for me to do when I am doing this work is to work with the energy in a heart-centered way. I'm so grateful for the highest and best experiences for each of my clients, as well as for myself. It truly brings me joy, when seeing the results of this alternative healing.

Finding A Good Healer

If you are looking to indulge in alternative medicine, your best bet in finding a good healer is by word of mouth. There are all different types of healers and some are educated, and some are self-taught. Keep in mind though, that each state has their own laws when referring to licenses and certifications. I have worked with and met many on both sides of the fence and they are very capable. So do your homework by consulting holistic journals in wholistic stores, alternative medicine wellness centers or credible alternative medicine educational programs. Make sure to ask all the questions you need, to feel comfortable with the best choice for you. While researching the degrees or certifications they have, remember to let your heart lead you to your healer.

There are Naturopaths, Healing Touch Practitioners, Acupuncturists, Aromatherapists, Herbalists, Reiki Practitioners and etc. When all else fails pick up some books or search credible internet sources for what you need.

Healing Both Bodies

Yes, you have two bodies, your physical body and your energetic body (chakra, aura, subtle body, etc). Most can't see energy with the untrained eye, but everyone can feel it. Everyone is radiating energy into the world all the time. To keep it simple, we all are made up of seven spinning wheels of energy. Those wheels are like whirlpools or vortexes called chakras. Your chakras can be opened or closed (blocked), just like the door to your home. Through energy work, you can elevate your level of energy and strengthen your own intuition for self-healing and clearing energy blockages. Blocked energy, purposely neglected, results in self-sabotage and steadily moves us into undesirable life experiences.

We have the power to self-heal our energy by unblocking it and clearing out the pain, hurt, and fear from our Chakras. We can then fill them with balance, peace, and joy.

Depending on the Chakra that is closed or blocked, this will have an impact on our mood and health. These energy centers bring us the truth about what is truly going on within our mind, body and spirit. But that's what self-healing and self-care are all about! They're about bringing the balance of your energies back and helping your mind, body, and spirit work in harmony in order to effect the positive changes in your life that you want to see.

The kind of energy you emanate can affect your life and also the lives of those around you. It creates a ripple effect, if you will. Whether you are conscious of it or not, you make a decision every day about the kind of energy you will radiate into the world. With self-care, you can choose free-flowing energy with positive results that not only improve your life, but also help boost others, as well.

This is not about religion! This is about being mindful within yourself, connecting with self and the highest and best part of you as you self-heal. For some, the highest and best part of us is our Higher Power, and for others it may be themselves. It's not my place to judge. But if you want more information, you can find countless more resources digitally or in your local library.

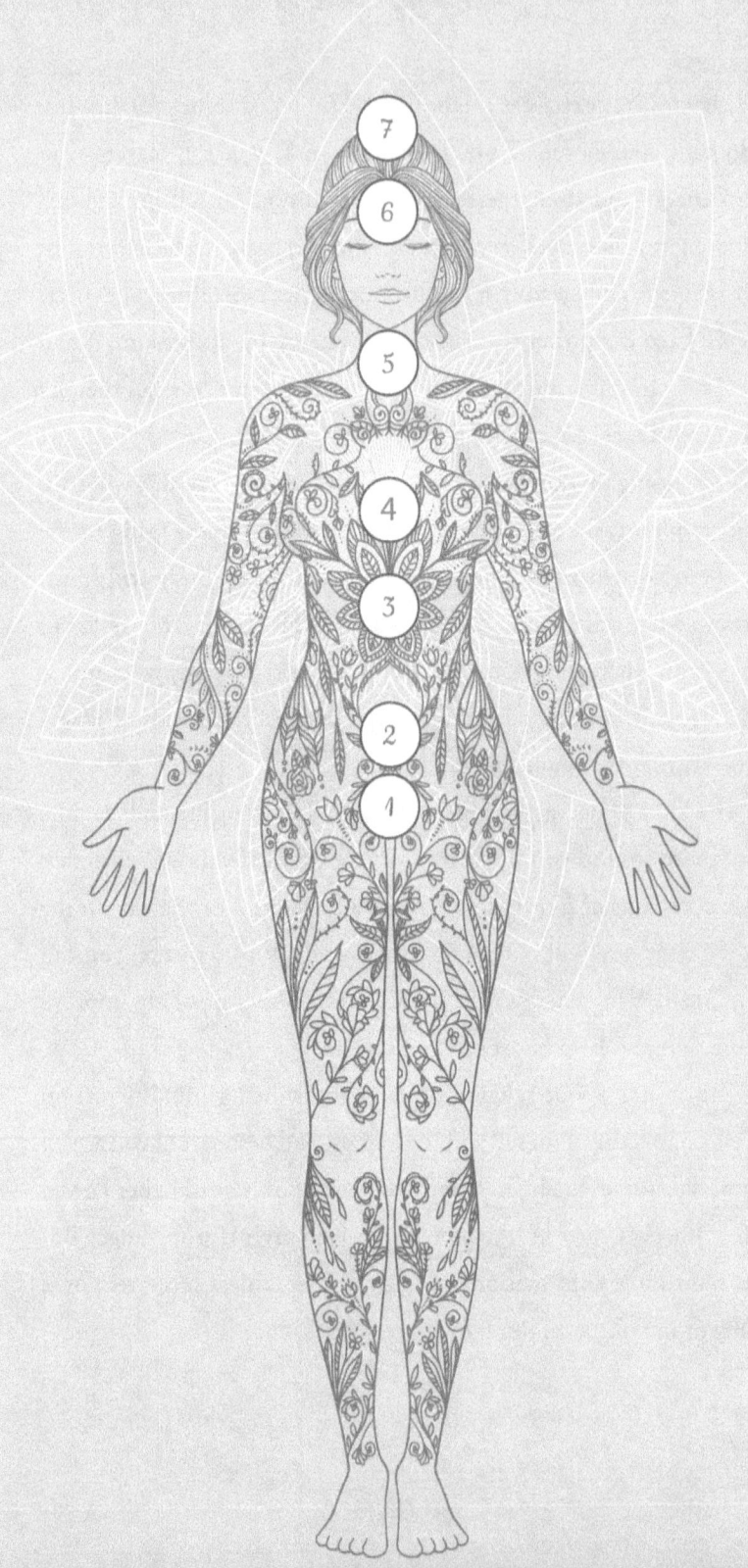

Chakra Healing Chart

⑦ **CROWN CHAKRA - ENLIGHTENMENT**
Associations: Affects inner and outer beauty, our connection to spirituality and pure bliss.
Color · Violet · I Know

⑥ **BROW CHAKRA - WISDOM**
Associated with intuition, imagination, wisdom and the ability to think and make decisions.
Color · Indigo · I See

⑤ **THROAT CHAKRA - TRUTH**
Affects communication, self-expression of feelings and the truth.
Color · Blue · I Speak

④ **HEART CHAKRA - LOVE**
Associated with love, joy and inner peace
Color · Green · I Love

③ **SOLAR PLEXUS CHAKRA — WILL POWER**
Associations are self-worth, self-confidence and self-esteem.
Color · Yellow · I Do

② **SACRAL CHAKRA - CREATIVITY**
Associated with a sense of abundance, well-being, pleasure, and sexuality.
Color · Orange · I Feel

① **ROOT CHAKRA — BASIC TRUST**
Associated with survival issues, trusting in the flow of life & will to live.
Color • Red • I Am

Rising to a Higher Level of Wellness

There are so many ways to raise the energetic vibrations within and around you with rest and relaxation, essential oils, music and eating the right foods and drinking the right liquids. The higher your energy vibration, the better you feel. It definitely starts with what we eat and how we eat. Do your own research on what works best for you. For me, I love Dr. Sebi's philosophy regarding eating energetic foods and an alkaline based diet. In addition, when I'm nourishing my body with plant-based foods, the unhealthy craving decreases significantly. I crave sugar much less and simply can't resist my fruits, vegetables and water. Drinking lots and lots of water, not only keeps me energized but it also keeps me feeling less sluggish and tired. Our bodies heal itself when we fall and scrape our knee, right? Well, the same is going on inside of us. Our body is healing itself every day, and how effective the results are from healthy eating habits, will be based on our food choices, exercising, de-stressing, and resting. Being in bed by 8 or 9 pm, gives my mind and body the preparation to settle down for rest and relaxation to fall asleep. It also promotes sleep by 10 pm when I'm shooting for an 8-hour nights' rest. Here are some of the foods and drinks that I love to eat to keep me healthy, and things I have cut out, in no particular order: Out: No chicken, no pork, no turkey, no milk, no red meat, no white sugar In: Blue Berries, Watercress, Seeded Grapes, Zucchini, Bananas, Olives, Apples, Bell Peppers, Limes, Strawberries, Onions, Mangos, Kale, Raspberries, Cucumbers, Cantaloupe, Avocados, Cherries, Seeded Melon, Arugula, Seeded Raisins, Chamomile tea, Ginger Tea, Fennel Tea and Raspberry Tea, and grapeseed oil for cooking and Olive Oil for salad dressings. By the way, if you're thinking "Wow, that's all she eats!", remember this is not about me… It took me watching a documentary called "What the Health" on Netflix to get me where I am. So, follow your own process, and do what works for you.

If you decide to indulge in your favorite dessert every now and then, no one, specifically me, is going to come hunt you down and pry it out of that death grip of yours. Especially since there is a strong possibility that I am probably doing the same. LOL! I refuse to beat myself up about it, and neither should you! Being gentle with yourself is also key when we are eating what we are supposed to eat and when we're not.

Essential Oils

[Disclaimer, this is for informational purposes only; it is not intended as medical instruction.]

Using the essential oils is another great way to support your physical body and energetic body (your chakras, aura, the subtle bodies) by harmonizing your energy. Simply put, your entire body can be moved to a more relaxing, de-stressed state just by dabbing your chakra or rubbing the oil in your hands while inhaling to make a connection between the oil and the energy centers. I've read an article or two regarding the use of aromatherapy during the recovery of substance abuse. Personally though, aromatherapy, art therapy and music therapy are all additional remedies that I've used for my mental health recovery (major depressive disorder, PTSD, Anxiety, etc.). It makes a whole lot of sense, when I think about how I feel after walking thru some tantalizing aroma's coming from my mom's kitchen; verses how I feel when I'm passing the roadkill of a dead skunk on the freeway. I'm sure you will agree, that both will put you in two totally different mind frames.

The oils listed are natural healing properties, just as Aloe Vera or eucalyptus plants, assist with healing us. I have put together a chart for essential oils so that you can research which of these fragrances will work best for your own self-healing and self-care needs. It's not a one size fits all approach. So do your homework!

Essential Oil Chart

Crown Chakra – Top of the Head
Incense • Rosewood

Brow Chakra – Middle of the Forehead
Violet · Lemongrass · Cajeput

Throat Chakra - Larynx
Eucalyptus · Peppermint · Camphor

Heart Chakra – Center of the Chest
Tarragon · Rose · Jasmine

Solar Plexus Chakra – Above the Navel
Chamomile • Anise • Lemon • Lavender

Sacral Chakra – Below the Navel
Pepper · Sandalwood · Myrrh · Bitter Orange

Root Chakra – Base of the spine
(between the genitals)
Cypress · Cedar · Rosemary · Cloves · Vanilla

"The Healing Partner" Work

Affirmation

I choose the energy of love and self-healing.

Acknowledgment

Acknowledge the part of you that is holding on to that which does not serve your higher purpose, the part of you that wants and needs to embody loving and healing energy.

Attunement

Attune with each of your seven chakras. Opening, balancing, and clearing the blockages within all of your energy centers can move you to a path of healing in mind, body, and spirit as a whole. As with everything else, it is both a *choice* and an *effort* that results in action.

"The Healing Partner" Thoughts:

[Disclaimer, this is for informational purposes only; it is not intended as medical instruction.]

Try these healing activities as you learn more about chakra energy flow.

Try to sense each of the different chakras within your body. Start with the first chakra and go up through each of the energy centers in your body. At first you may not feel anything, or you may wonder if you are forcing yourself to feel something that isn't there. Don't worry about this. With a little practice, you will learn to sense each of your chakras and be able to feel them in your body. The first step to this, though, is just to start exploring. So, spend a few minutes just trying to feel the energy in each of these parts of the body. As you try to identify the energy centers, you can also reflect on the ideas listed in the Chakra Chart.

When you start to feel your chakras, the sensation you will have will likely be a warm, fuzzy sense in that center of energy. You've probably felt this in your heart at some point in your life, like when you're experiencing love. A similar kind of awareness is possible with the other energy centers in the body.

For a fun and informative challenge, see if your favorite color lines up with where your strength is—or what you yearn for more of.

Thoughts...

Final Thoughts

*"We all may have been a victim of circumstance
or a perpetrator of mistakes,
but it will never change our DNA, the color of our eyes,
or the Victor within.
We just have to move into who we've always been...
The Victor!
So, move, Victor, move!"
– PerCilla, "The Healing Partner"*

WE'VE covered a lot in this book, and I've shared some of my personal confessions, painful struggles, and lively personality. I'm optimistic that my words will inspire you to act, to make choices, and to do something to create positive changes within yourself that will ripple throughout the universe.

I hope you've found enough information, helpful anecdotes, and even some moments of humor to help guide you on your path to a brighter, healthier, more harmonious you. Make no mistake about it, we all may have been a victim of circumstance or a perpetrator of mistakes, but it never changes our DNA, the color of our eyes, or the "Victor" within us. We just have to clear out the rubbish in the stream and move into the person we've always been. Remember these two key words: "Move," and "victor!" So, move victor, move! As you move in the direction of your self-care and self-healing, know that it's a lot like a child forming in the womb. Pushing too soon and forcing these things into the world before they're ready isn't the best idea for a great birth. However, allow your intentions and goals to evolve and grow. Make space for patience and give your growth time to expand.

I want to reiterate that flowing through this information, instead of forcing it, will be key to your process. Learning to connect to your Higher Source or self through a practice of mindfulness and daily meditation will help significantly, also.

Many people advocate the practice of mindfulness and meditation to help with: anxiety from impatience, stress from judgmentalism, worry about the future, and depression from thinking about the past. These practices are like your safety net from all of that. I highly recommend them. Adding a safety net means you will have a more connected experience throughout the stages of your self-healing journey.

Don't overanalyze things that don't serve you well in getting the healing you need. Turning your focus to your Source and listening to your still, inner voice is the only thing you need to tap into your self-healing and self-care. I can't emphasize enough that this is not about religion. However, it can be a spiritual practice, if you choose.

For me, this is about putting a practice of peace, harmony, and love in place. It's one that has extended beyond my physical self, filled my void, and healed my pain through the loving energy that was given to it. But that is *me!*

For yourself, go ahead and use this knowledge the way you want and find most helpful. Break that highlighter out, bend some page corners, and flip back and forth to customize the information to fill the

I Am Healing - Final Thoughts

need for a "Self-Care Plan," as best fits *you*.

You matter here! Whether or not you're in a church, a mosque, a synagogue, a temple—if you're lying on your bed or sitting under your favorite willow tree on a bright sunny day—tap into your Source to connect with yourself; that is what's most important here.

That is the only determining factor for your highest and best good. When you learn to make that connection, it can help you to see your life from a different perspective—and from the most important perspective: the authentic you. So, take everything one day at a time; this is a lot of information, and you won't *get it* all in one day.

There's so much more I'd love to share with you about self-care and self-healing, energy medicine, and ways to brighten your inner light, but it would be difficult to put it all in one book. And just like you, I am learning more and more each day. Not just as an apprentice progressing into my practitionership, but also as a person, like you, staying in tune with my own self-healing.

Since there is so much more to learn and know about energy medicine (rather than just reading about it), better yet, why don't you book an in-person session or schedule a tele-wellness session with me on my website (see below). I also invite you to sign up for one of my health and wellness retreats or workshops.

Finally, there are also more treats from my heart to yours available on my social media and website! My site, www.PerCillaZeno.com is the hub of my in-person and online services. I love to help people, so I find joy sharing and interacting on my social media pages, because I want to spread the healing message far and wide.

I've dedicated my life to life's challenges to recovery, self-healing, self-care, energy medicine, and whole health wellness. Because I want to see everyone living a healthier, happier, and a more light-filled, authentic life, I wanted to reach inside myself and give a part of me that would heal apart of you. It's my hopes that my words have welcomed the self-love and self-healing you deserve. Together, we can spread love and light, and live in bliss, if we all reach inside ourselves and give the most authentic, highest and best part of us.

Thank you again for supporting our 501c nonprofit - That Zen Life Wellness, Foundation, Inc. with the purchase of this book. 100% of the proceeds, go to the nonprofit.

As a free gift please visit my webpage https://www.percillazeno.com/evaluation to receive a Free Chakra Evaluation. Find out which of your chakra's have the greatest influence and which of them are compromised.

I have also provided a list of Resources for lots of organizations that can assist with your life path.

This book is just one of the ways I'm bringing comfort to people in need, and I'd love to meet you in person, dear reader. I'd love to help you on your journey as your Healing Partner. Visit my online store for the I AM Healing: 7 Secrets to Wellness & Self-Care Journal and other Kool Stuff!

Thank you for reading this book. I hope you enjoyed it. You can view more of my work, and upcoming events on my social media.

Feel free to reach out to me. Sending you love and light. *Be Well! Rock On!*

PerCilla Zeno, "The Healing Partner"

Services & Merchandise

PerCillaZeno.com

TheHealingPartner.com

ZandZPublishing.com

ThatZenLife.org

Social Media

FB:/TheHealingPartnerWorldwide

FB:/ThatZenLifeWellnessNonProfit

IG: @TheHealingPartner

IG: @ThatZenLIfeNonProfit

TW: @PerCillaZeno

IN: @PerCillaZeno

#IAMHealing7Secrets

Acknowledgements

Special thanks to:

Thank you to Dobeir "Doe Bear" Rudolph and Kenya Watts, for the *branding* insights. Thank you Dobeir for helping with the name of the nonprofit. I am so grateful to have you both in my life.

And to my stylist, makeup artist and business enthusiast, Deja Rudolph — thank you for making me look beautiful and for connecting me with what was needed for me to move forward. What would I do without you?

All my siblings— for the divine in you. For the spirit that draws us together, sharing and caring for one another. As it should be. I am so grateful.

Renee, Carlene, and Claos— for locking my secrets away not only in your heads, but also in your hearts; for your friendship, for listening to me, crying with me, laughing with me, encouraging me, loving on me— and for being the roots beneath my tree of life.

Author and cousin Alicia Singleton—for always providing love, support, positivity, and wisdom without compromise. Thank you for giving me the wings needed to take flight on my writing journey. You are the best writing coach ever! Blessings, Love and Light to you always.

Dr. Harriette Barnes Parker and Dr. Huma Hyder—for your support, encouragement, and conversations in a safe place, just as therapy should be. Sometimes it didn't even seem like therapy. Thank you for that as well.

Simon Timm—for being more than an editor. For your friendship, kindness, and guidance. So happy that the universe allowed our paths to align. Thank you for believing in me and for the fire in your heart to see me WIN. I will forever be grateful. Sending you love, peace and joy always. Namaste my friend.

Claudia Rose, PhD. – Thank you for your open heart, your open mind and your willingness to listen to spirit speak and sharing the outcome with the world and most of all thank you for sharing your kindness, your beautifully deep conversations, your laughs and your divine friendship with me. I am Humbled and Grateful. Love & Light to you always.

Deva Premal and Miten—thank you for staying true to who you are. I'm so grateful that your music was the conduit for Spirit to speak to me in a way that I could hear and evolve.

To the women who gave their consent to share their stories anonymously, you are healers. I am inspired by your strength and your courage. I thank you so much for sharing your stories in a selfless manner to help others heal. Know that your story will be a positive ripple effect throughout the Universe. I am so grateful. Thank you. WE DID IT!

Thank you to my energy medicine instructors: Marilyn Stulb, Lynne Whitlock, and many more. Without your instruction, I would not have made it were I am thus far. Thank you.

To my biological father for being a part of the reason for my existence. I thank you for the lessons you taught me that has helped me grow. I would not be who I am without them. I speak to the five-year-old boy in you and say he has always been good and *is* good. I speak to the man in you and say: "The opportunity to heal lies before us daily, despite our tough experiences, mistakes, and conscious faults. Daily we can choose to acknowledge and evolve. I send you love, peace, light, and forgiveness."

Notes

Notes

Notes

Notes

Notes

Notes

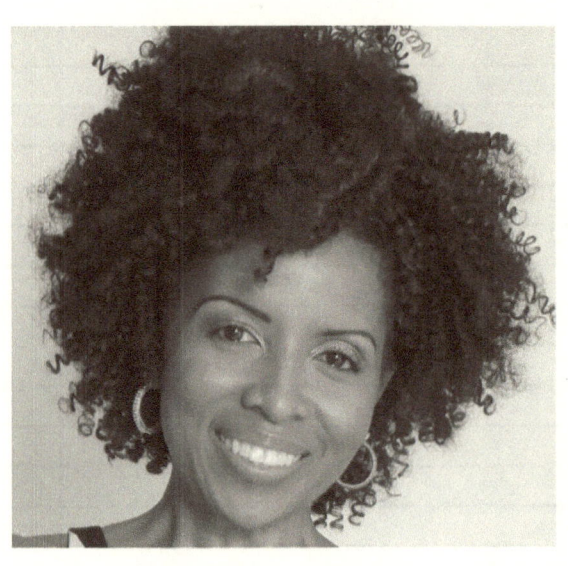

About the Author

"A healer is not a person you go to for healing, it's a person who trigger's within you your own ability to heal."

- Unknown

PERCILLA Zeno was born in Washington, DC, and reared in Southeast San Diego, CA. She is an energetic voice in our time—sharing her moxie, wit, and wisdom as an authentic motivational speaker/educator, prolific healer/entrepreneur, and now dynamic published author. Her mantra is simple: "Let go, clear your fear, and flow forward, while filling the undesirable spaces in your life with positively everything you need." When not healing herself or her clients with Energy Medicine, she can be found dancing, traveling, meditating, or loving on her children and husband, Luis. She lives in Hampton Roads, Virginia.

Executive Partner of her own publishing company, among other enterprises, PerCilla is a go-getter extraordinaire who passionately empowers others to uncover their best self—their I Am—and rise from trapped to transcendent!

Friends and colleagues call her a "force of nature." Not one to waste energy, she's given back to her community not just as a member of the Order of The Eastern Star® but also in the Commonwealth of Virginia, as the president of the nonprofit That Zen Life Wellness Foundation,

Inc. As a Community Health Worker who is State Board Certified in the specialization of Peer Recovery Support and Community Health, she's also a Healing Touch Practitioner Apprentice and holds 4 of the 5 certifications in Healing Touch Therapy and is working on her 5th and last certification as a practitioner in Energy Medicine. The birth of her 5 children, marrying the love of her life, and supporting others in their well-being are just a few of the highlights that keep her driven. PerCilla's mentorship through retreats, support via one-on-ones, and giving back to the mental health, recovery, and whole health community, using alternative medicine or peer recovery support is her passion. PerCilla also enjoys dancing, outdoor meditation, traveling and being a foodie.

* *

"I am a healer. I have many gifts that I did not ask for but I'm so grateful to use them to help others. They came to me during a time I did not feel I was worthy of them. Writing this book, help me understand that daily I may fall short and in the same turn, daily I am worthy. We are all healers when we take the time to trigger within someone's ability to heal. Every person is different. However, it can happen with a conversation, a therapy session, a hug, an apology, an understanding, and a healing touch with simple humility, empathy, love, gratitude, kindness and most importantly with the absence of EGO." PerCilla, The Healing Partner

Resources

THE resources compiled in this list are hotlines, websites and phone numbers provided for (3) purposes. It is to provide:

◊ the information needed to those who can get it out or those who can use it themselves.

◊ a list of organizations you may want to become apart of and give back to.

◊ a plethora of options and outlets before anyone decides to give up. And if you are one of those people reading this… Know that some have been where you are.

So just like us, someone else has experienced it, that someone else has gotten through it and that someone one else has risen from it. Just as my full knowledge has brought me to being a published author, certifications in healing, health, and wellness know that you have a purpose too! All these resources, to the best of my knowledge are up-to-date. But, keep in mind that as time goes on things change. So if you run into any challenges, *google it!*

CRISIS HOTLINES

National Suicide Prevention Lifeline
Website: http://www.suicidepreventionlifeline.org/
Description: This is a confidential, toll-free, 24-hour suicide prevention hotline. Call 1-800-273-TALK to receive counseling and local referrals.

National Domestic Violence Hotline
Website: http://www.thehotline.org/
Description: The National Domestic Violence Hotline provides 24/7 counseling and support to victims of domestic violence and abuse at 1-800-799-SAFE (7233).

American Social Health Association:
Sexually Transmitted Disease Hotline - 1-800-227-8922

Veterans Crisis Line
Website: http://www.veteranscrisisline.net/
Description: The Veterans Crisis Line provides confidential help for veterans and their families at
1-800-273-8255.

Mental Health Project
Website: http://smhp.psych.ucla.edu/hotline.htm
Description: UCLA's School Mental Health Project compiled a list of hotlines that are useful for school practitioners.

Child Help USA National Child Abuse hotline
http://www.childhelp.org/resources/

Safe Horizon

Website: http://www.safehorizon.org

Description: Sexual assault prevention and awareness organization Safe Horizon provides a hotline for domestic violence victims, sexual assault victims and crime victims to receive 24/7 free crisis counseling and safety planning. - 1- 800-621-HOPE (4673).

Getting Help

That Zen Life Wellness Foundation, Inc. - Whole Health & Peer Recovery Support Services

Website: http://www.ThatZenLife.org

Our mission is to promote nonclinical whole health wellness and recovery support. We do this by offering social reconnection events, Text and tele-wellness services, e-Peer Recovery Support, educational tools and resources, no insurance required. We are open to servicing veterans and their spouses, single and/or grieving parents, returning citizens, LGBTQ community and any adult in recovery of trauma, mental health, drug or alcohol challenges. We carry out that mission through an intentional, nonjudgmental, accepting, and calming way. (757) 932 – 5663 (Voice / Text)

Substance Abuse and Mental Health Services Administration

Website: http://findtreatment.samhsa.gov/

Description: This site is a SAMHSA's behavioral treatment services locator.

McShin Foundation
Website: https://www. mcshin.org

Description: The McShin Foundation is a Recovery Community Organization (RCO). An RCO is defined in-part as having resources such as: Halfway Houses, Transitional Recovery Houses, Opiate Detox, and being connected with alcohol and drug rehabs, substance abuse treatment and aftercare. We offer a social model recovery program that implements Peer-to-peer delivered Recovery Support Services (PRSS).

The Healing Touch
http://hticp.com/content_assets/docs/current/Facilities_Using_Healing_Touch_Nov_2016.pdf

Find a Therapist

Website: https://www.psychologytoday.com/us/therapists

Description: The Find a Therapist service from Psychology Today helps users find mental health professionals in their area.

American Psychological Association Help Center
Website: https://www.apa.org/helpcenter/index.aspx

Description: The American Psychological Association's Help Center contains a Find a Psychologist directory and help resources in the areas of work and school, family and relationships, health and emotional wellness, disasters and terrorism, and managed care and health insurance

Anxiety, OCD, PTSD and Depression

Anxiety and Depression Association of America

Website: https://adaa.org/living-with-anxiety

Description: The Anxiety and Depression Association of America raises public and professional awareness, promotes research advancement and provides referrals for children and adults with anxiety, depression, obsessive compulsive disorder, post-traumatic stress disorders and related disorders. The website provides information about these conditions, their treatment and resources for professionals.

Anxiety Disorder Resource Center

Website: http://www.adaa.org/living-with-anxiety

Description: The American Academy of Child & Adolescent Psychiatry's Anxiety Disorder Resource Center contains a glossary of symptoms and mental illnesses, a child and adolescent psychiatrist finder, facts and resources for families and youth suffering from anxiety and anxiety-related disorders.

Freedom from Fear

Website: http://www.freedomfromfear.org/

Description: This is the website of the nonprofit advocacy organization Freedom from Fear. It contains a wealth of research-based information and treatment referrals for anxiety and depression.

American Psychological Association

Website: https://www.apa.org

Description: This is the official website of the American Psychological Association, the largest professional psychology association in the country. It's made up of more than 130,000 clinicians, researchers, consultants, educators and students.

American Psychiatric Association

Website: http://www.psych.org/

Description: This is the official website of the American Psychiatric Association, the largest psychiatric organization in the world. It's made up of more than 35,000 member psychiatrists.

Substance Abuse

Substance Abuse and Mental Health Services Administration

Website: http://www.samhsa.gov/

Description: The Substance Abuse and Mental Health Services Administration, the U.S. Department of Health and Human Services agency on behavioral health, runs several mental health campaigns and has information on health reform for providers, families and individuals. SAMHSA also has a helpful online behavioral treatment services locator.

National Help Line - 1-800-662-HELP (4357)

Additional Substance Abuse Hotlines
Al-Anon for Families of Alcoholics - (888) 425-2666 Alcohol & Drug Abuse Hotline - 1-800-729-6686 Cocaine Anonymous - (800) 347-8998

Families Anonymous - (800) 736-9805

National Council on Alcoholism and Drug Dependence Hopeline - (800) 622-2255

Military/Veterans

Veterans Affairs
Website: http://www.mentalhealth.va.gov/

Description: The U.S. Department of Veterans Affairs website hosts screening tools, a veterans crisis line and a guide to mental health conditions that often plague veterans.

National Association on Mental Illness
Website: https://www.nami.org/veterans

Description: The National Association on Mental Illness has a Veterans & Military Resource Center, which is home to online discussion groups, information about veteran mental illnesses and treatments. It includes information about advocacy for active-duty members, returning veterans, veteran families, veterans in recovery, veterans looking for work, mental health providers, college faculty members and women veterans.

Military Pathways
Website: https://www.militarymentalhealth.org/

Description: Military Pathways is a site created by Screening for Mental Health and the Department of Defense that allows military members and their families to take free, anonymous mental health or alcohol self-assessments. Completion of the assessment directs users to referral information for Department of Defense and Veterans Affairs services.

Lesbian, gay, bisexual and transgender

National Alliance on Mental Illness
Website: https://www.cdc.gov/lgbthealth/index.htm

Description: The National Alliance on Mental Illness GLBT resources page contains articles, videos, publications, research and links to prominent organizations about GLBT mental health.

GLBT National Help Center
Website: http://www.glbtnationalhelpcenter.org/

Description: The GLBT National Help Center provides an online peer-support chat as well as free, confidential counseling over the phone for the GLBT community.

The Trevor Project
Website: http://www.thetrevorproject.org/

Description: The creators of the Oscar-winning short film "Trevor" founded The Trevor Project. The organization provides suicide prevention and crisis intervention for LGBTQ youth between the ages of 13 and 24.

Help Center on Sexual Orientation

Website: http://www.apa.org/helpcenter/sexual-orientation.aspx

Description: The American Psychological Association's Help Center on Sexual Orientation's website provides research and information on mental health issues surrounding sexual orientation.

Seniors

National Institutes of Health

Website: https://www.nia.nih.gov/health

Description: The National Institutes of Health provides this online index of information, videos and training tools about senior health, including mental health and wellness.

National Council on Aging

Website: https://www.ncoa.org/center-for-healthy-aging/behavioral-health/

Description: The National Council on Aging promotes programs that help seniors cope with mental health issues like depression, anxiety, addiction and more.

National Association of Mental Illness

Website: https://www.nami.org/

Description: The National Association of Mental Illness is the largest nationwide mental health advocacy grassroots organization with hundreds of state organizations, affiliates and volunteers. It is a hub for support groups, free education, raising awareness and building community.

Mental Health Resources, Inc.
Website: http://www.mhresources.org/

Description: This nonprofit provides community-based mental health services to adults, especially those suffering medical, social or substance-related comorbidities.

American Psychiatry Association
Website: http://www.psychiatry.org/mental-health/ _

Description: The American Psychiatry Association is the largest professional membership organization of psychiatrists in the world. The APA website hosts "Let's Talk Facts" brochures on a range of illnesses, professional resources for psychiatrists, psychiatric residents and medical students. It publishes up-to-date news, research, government policies and developments in psychiatry.

Screening for Mental Health
Website: http://www.mentalhealthscreening.org/

Description: Providing schools, workplaces, colleges, and communities the tools to address mental health issues, substance use, and suicide risk.

I Am Healing - Resources

School and College Students

The Jed Foundation

Website: http://www.jedfoundation.org/

Description: The Jed Foundation is an organization committed to the mental and emotional health of college students and preventing suicide among this population. The foundation runs several free online self-assessment and resource programs for students and campuses. It offers training tools for campus professionals to improve their mental health services for students.

ULifeline

Website: http://www.ulifeline.org/

Description: A project of the Jed Foundation that provides a free, confidential online resource about emotional health to more than 1,500 colleges and universities.

LawLifeline

Website: http://www.lawlifeline.org

Description: LawLifeline is a combined project of the Jed Foundation and Dave Nee Foundation. It is a free, anonymous and confidential online resource for law school students to seek out information about depression, anxiety, suicide, stress and self-harm.

Healing Private Wounds

Healing Private Wounds is a non-profit outreach ministry with two main focuses: to help victims and families traumatized by sexual abuse to find healing and peace and to provide education and increase awareness of sexual abuse to help stop sexual crimes in our homes and communities.

http://www.healingprivatewounds.org

WOMEN

Office on Women's Health
Website: https://www.womenshealth.gov/mental-health/resources/

Description: The Office on Women's Health of the U.S. Department of Health and Human Services provides access to research, publications, Surgeon General Reports and general information for women's mental health issues. This includes problems related to pregnancy and conception, menstruation, menopause, women veterans, suicide prevention and mental illnesses.

World Health Organization
Website: https://www.who.int/mental_health/prevention/

Description: The World Health Organization website contains a section on global mental health as it relates to issues of gender and gender disparity.

MINORITY

Office of Minority Health
Website: http://minorityhealth.hhs.gov/templates/browse.aspx?lvl=2&lvlID=26

Description: The U.S. Department of Health and Human Services Office of Minority Health website provides statistics, news and treatment information.

I Am Healing - Resources

Support

Mental Health America

Website: http://www.mentalhealthamerica.net/

Description: Mental Health America is a community-based network with 240 nationwide affiliates that provide services such as counseling referrals, support and finding housing for the homeless.

National Council for Behavioral Health

Website: http://www.thenationalcouncil.org/

Description: The National Council for Behavioral Health is a collective of more than 2,000 member mental health and substance abuse treatment organizations. The National Council is known for creating Mental Health First Aid, a public education initiative consisting of an eight-hour course that provides participants with a crash course in understanding mental illness risk factors, impacts and treatments. It is aimed at increasing early detection and intervention.

Eating Disorders

National Eating Disorders Association

Website: https://www.nationaleatingdisorders.org

Description: The National Eating Disorders Association is a nonprofit supporting people with eating disorders and their families. It provides an information and referral helpline, extensive information about eating disorder prevention, treatment and recovery, as well as handouts and toolkits for parents, coaches and educators, and forums for discussion and stories of recovery. The website is also available in Spanish.

Proud2Bme

Website: http://proud2bme.org/

Description: An online community for teens that encourage healthy body image.

Bipolar

Depression and Bipolar Support Alliance

Website: http://www.dbsalliance.org/

Description: The Depression and Bipolar Support Alliance is a national peer-led organization run by individuals with depression and bipolar disorder. It provides support groups, peer specialist training, wellness tools, research, podcasts, brochures, publications and information for clinicians.

The Balanced Mind

Website: http://www.thebalancedmind.org/ _

Description: The Balanced Mind, a parent network run by the Depression and Bipolar Support Alliance, provides support and guidance to parents raising children with mood disorders.

www.ingramcontent.com/pod-product-compliance
Lightning Source LLC
Chambersburg PA
CBHW020418080526
44584CB00014B/1383